Mainstreaming HIV/AIDS in Development and Humanitarian Programmes

ActionAid, Oxfam GB, and Save the Children UK

ActionAid is a partnership of people who are fighting for a better world – a world without poverty. As one of the UK's largest development agencies, ActionAid works in over 35 countries in Africa, Asia, Latin America, and the Caribbean, listening to, learning from, and working in partnership with more than nine million of the world's poorest people.
ActionAid, Hamlyn House, Macdonald Road, London N19 5PG, UK
www.actionaid.org

Oxfam GB, founded in 1942, is a development, humanitarian, and campaigning agency dedicated to finding lasting solutions to poverty and suffering around the world. Oxfam believes that every human being is entitled to a life of dignity and opportunity, and it works with others worldwide to make this become a reality. Oxfam GB is a member of Oxfam International, a confederation of 12 agencies which share a commitment to working for an end to injustice and poverty – both in long-term development work and at times of crisis.
Oxfam GB, Oxfam House, 274 Banbury Road, Oxford, OX2 7DZ, UK
www.oxfam.org.uk
www.oxfam.org.uk/publications

Save the Children is the UK's leading international children's charity, working to create a better future for children. It is a member of the International Save the Children Alliance, which is active in over 100 countries worldwide. Drawing on this practical experience, Save the Children also seeks to influence policy and practice to achieve lasting benefits for children within their communities. In all its work, Save the Children endeavours to make children's rights a reality.
Save the Children UK, 1 St John's Lane, London EC1M 4AR, UK
www.savethechildren.org.uk

Mainstreaming HIV/AIDS in Development and Humanitarian Programmes

Sue Holden

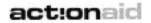

Oxfam

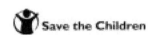

Practical Action Publishing Ltd
25 Albert Street, Rugby, CV21 2SD, Warwickshire, UK
www.practicalactionpublishing.org

First published by Oxfam GB in association with ActionAid and Save the
Children UK in 2004
Reprinted by Practical Action Publishing

© Oxfam GB 2004

Oxfam GB is registered as a charity in England and Wales (no. 202918) and
Scotland (SCO 039042).
Oxfam GB is a member of Oxfam International.

Paperback ISBN: 978-0-85598-530-1
PDF ISBN: 9780855987909
Book DOI: http://dx.doi.org/10.3362/9780855987909

A catalogue record for this publication is available from the British Library.

Contents

List of figures

List of tables

Acknowledgements

I would like to thank Susan Amoaten, Ruth Mkhwanazi Bechtel, Marjan Besuijen, and Harriet Kivumbi Nkalubo for their very useful comments on the draft text for this book. I must also acknowledge Catherine Robinson's contribution as an excellent and most amiable editor.

Many people contributed to *AIDS on the Agenda*, and so, indirectly, to this book. I am grateful to them all:

John Abuya, Santos Alfredo, Patience Alidri, Susan Amoaten, Craig Ash, Ellen Bajenja, Jacqueline Bataringaya, Roxanne Bazergan, Abeba Bekele, Vera Bensmann, Renuka Bery, Saida Bogere, Tania Boler, Samuel Braimah, Sr Carol Breslin, Ned Breslin, Audace Buderi, Rogers Bulsuwa, Kate Butcher, Dawn Cavanagh, Sifiso Chikandi, Joe Collins, Chris Desmond, Jill Donahue, Michael Drinkwater, Janet Duffield, Lyn Elliott, Helen Elsey, Tabitha Elwes, Andrew Fitzgibbon, Josef Gardiner, Afonsina Gonzaga, Angela Hadjipateras, Jim Henry, Alexander Heroys, Fortunate Hofisi, Ulli Huber, Liz Hughes, Rick James, Phoebe Kajubi, Kristin Kalla, Dinah Kasangaki, Juma Kariburyo, Lawrence Khonyongwa, Kate Kilpatrick, Sarah Lee, Rachel MacCarthy, Ryann Manning, David Mawejje, Rosemarie McNairn, John Mkwere, Duduzile Moyo, Dan Mullins, Carmen Murguia, Hussein Mursal, Tom Muzoora, Kondwani Mwangulube, Dennis Nduhura, Stella Neema, Jack van Niftrick, Josephine Niyonkuru, Nellie Nyang'wa, Grace Odolot, Akua Ofori-Asumadu, Joseph Okello, Alfred Okema, Akua Kwateng-Addo, Nick Osborne, Sam Page, Bill Rau, Jenny Rawden, Linnea Renton, Jose Sluijs, Rose Smart, Ann Smith, Mohga Kamal-Smith, Hilary Standing, Woldemedhin Tekletsadik, Bridgette Thorold, Daphne Topouzis, Dolar Vasani, Rachel Waterhouse, Douglas Webb, Jo White, and Alan Whiteside.

The research on which this book is based, and the costs of the production of the book, were funded by a generous grant from the United Kingdom Department for International Development (DFID), for the benefit of developing countries. The views expressed are not necessarily those of the UK government, and do not necessarily reflect the policy of DFID.

Sue Holden
Lancaster, April 2004

Abbreviations

AIDS   Acquired Immune Deficiency Syndrome

ASO   AIDS support organisation

CBO   community-based organisation

FAO   Food and Agriculture Organisation of the United Nations

GB   Great Britain

GIPA   Greater Involvement of People with AIDS

HIV   Human Immunodeficiency Virus

NGO   non-government organisation

STI   sexually transmitted infection

TB   tuberculosis

UNAIDS   The Joint United Nations Programme on HIV/AIDS

UNDP   United Nations Development Programme

UNHCR   United Nations High Commissioner for Refugees

Glossary

Please note that there are separate entries for words or phrases printed in italics.

AIDS support organisations	Organisations dedicated to, or working with a primary focus on, *AIDS work*, including prevention, care, and treatment.
AIDS work	Work which is directly focused on AIDS prevention, or care, treatment, or support for people infected with HIV. AIDS work is distinct from, and implemented separately from, other development and humanitarian work. For example, educational initiatives to change behaviour, and home-based care programmes.
antiretroviral therapies	Combinations of drugs which act on HIV to delay or reverse the onset of AIDS, enabling people who are infected with HIV to live longer and with a better quality of life.
endemic	(Describing a disease or infection): continuously prevalent in a particular location, community, or population.
epidemic	A widespread outbreak of a disease or infection within a population.
food security	Access to sufficient and sustainable supplies of food to meet dietary needs for an active and healthy life.
gender	Refers to socially determined differences between men's and women's roles, behaviours, and opportunities, rather than biological differences between the two sexes.

HIV-positive	Infected with HIV (which, when it enters someone's blood, stimulates the development of antibodies, which can be detected by tests; so a person who is infected with HIV is said to be HIV (antibody) positive, HIV-positive, or HIV+). HIV gradually destroys the *immune system*, leaving the person *susceptible* to other infections.
HIV prevalence	The proportion of people in a population who are *HIV-positive* at a given time – usually measured as a proportion of adults aged 15–49.
immune system	The body's means of resisting infection.
integrated AIDS work	*AIDS work* which is carried out as part of development and humanitarian work. The focus is on direct prevention, care, treatment, or support, but the work is conducted in conjunction with, and linked to, other projects, or within wider programmes. For example, HIV prevention as part of broader health-promotion programmes, or treatment as part of wider health services.
livelihood	Means of living or supporting oneself or one's household, such as farming, trading, providing services, salaried employment, or combinations of various kinds of work.
mainstreaming HIV/ AIDS internally	Changing policy and practice in order to reduce the organisation's *susceptibility to HIV infection* and its *vulnerability to the impacts of AIDS*. The focus is on HIV/AIDS and the organisation. It has two elements: *AIDS work* with staff, such as prevention and treatment; and modifying the ways in which the organisation functions; for example, changes in workforce planning and budgeting.
mainstreaming HIV/ AIDS externally	Adapting development and humanitarian programme work in order to take into account *susceptibility to HIV transmission* and *vulnerability to the impacts of AIDS*. The focus is on core programme work in the changing context created by HIV/AIDS. For example, an agricultural project which is adjusted to the needs of vulnerable households in an AIDS-affected community.

modes of HIV transmission	The ways in which HIV may be passed from one infected person to another: during *unsafe sex*, through *unsafe medical procedures*, through *other unsafe practices*, and from mother to child during pregnancy, childbirth, and breastfeeding.
opportunistic infections	Parasitic, bacterial, viral, and fungal infections which take hold when someone's *immune system* is weakened. Common infections include tuberculosis, thrush, shingles, meningitis, and pneumonia. They may resist treatment, or they may seem to be cured but later they recur. People with HIV are also prone to developing cancers, including those caused by viruses and cancers of the *immune system*.
other unsafe practices	Non-medical practices in which equipment is used to cut or pierce the skin of more than one person without being adequately sterilised or disinfected to prevent HIV transmission. Such practices include injecting drugs, decorating the body with tattoos or scars, and circumcision.
pandemic	A widespread outbreak of a disease or infection affecting the population of a wide area of the world.
positive living	A concept developed by people living with HIV infection who acknowledge that they have HIV; try to eat a well-balanced diet; take exercise, while also getting rest and avoiding stress; abstain from sexual activity, or practise *safer sex*; get treatment for *opportunistic infections;* and attend to their mental and spiritual health. Positive living may also embrace preparing for death, for example by making a will, and making arrangements for dependants.
productive assets	Possessions which are used to generate income or to grow food, such as land; tools and equipment; and animals which are used in farming or business.
protective assets	Money which a household can spend in times of need, and possessions that it can sell, while

protecting its *productive assets* and so its ability to grow food or to generate income. For example, non-productive items such as jewellery, or equipment such as a radio.

safer sex	Sexual activities which reduce or prevent the exchange of body fluids that can transmit HIV (blood, semen, pre-ejaculatory fluid, and vaginal fluid), by using barriers such as condoms, or engaging in sexual practices in which those fluids are not exchanged.
sexual and gender-based violence	Includes physical, sexual, and psychological abuse, such as non-consenting sexual acts, sex with a minor, rape, female genital mutilation, forced marriage, domestic abuse, forced prostitution, and sexual harassment.
susceptibility to HIV infection	Likelihood of becoming infected by HIV. The word applies both to individuals and to groups of people; so it can refer to the probability of an organisation experiencing HIV infection among its employees, or the likelihood of a society experiencing an HIV *epidemic*. Susceptibility is determined by the economic and social character of a society, relationships between groups, *livelihood* strategies, culture, and balance of power (particularly with regard to *gender*).
unsafe medical procedures	Practices involving the use of blood or blood products or organs contaminated with HIV.
unsafe sex	Practices involving the exchange of body fluids that can transmit HIV (blood, semen, pre-ejaculatory fluid, and vaginal fluid) from an infected person to a partner during vaginal, anal, or (rarely) oral sex.
vulnerability to the impacts of AIDS	Openness to negative consequences as a result of AIDS. Refers to the likelihood of suffering harm from the effects of sickness and death due to AIDS. Can be applied to individuals, or to groups of people such as households, organisations, or societies. Vulnerability is made worse by poverty, fragmented social and family structures, and *gender* inequality.

Part 1 | The case for mainstreaming HIV/AIDS

1 | Introduction

AIDS depends for its success on the failures of development. If the world was a fairer place, if opportunities for men and women were equal, if everyone was well nourished, good public services were the norm, and conflict was a rarity, then HIV (Human Immunodeficiency Virus) would not have spread to its current extent, nor would the impacts of AIDS (Acquired Immune Deficiency Syndrome) be as great. We now know that the spread of HIV and the effects of AIDS are closely linked to development problems such as poverty and gender inequality. Development and humanitarian agencies should be doing more to respond to the challenges posed by HIV/AIDS. This book suggests a way in which they can do so through their existing work without necessarily establishing special programmes of HIV prevention or AIDS care.

This book is a shorter, simplified version of *AIDS on the Agenda* (Holden 2003), a book which can be ordered from Oxfam GB, or downloaded for free from http://www.oxfam.org.uk/what_we_do/issues/hivaids/aidsagenda.htm. The ideas in the two books are the same; but this version, we hope, is accessible to a wider range of readers: those who actually do development and humanitarian work, in addition to those who manage it and fund it. Unlike *AIDS on the Agenda*, this book does not feature quotations and case studies; instead it presents general lessons learned – mainly from the experiences of non-government and community-based organisations (NGOs and CBOs) working in the parts of Africa that are worst affected by HIV/AIDS.

AIDS has changed the world. This book is about the changes that we need to make in order to do effective development and humanitarian work in a world of AIDS.

What this book contains

Part 1 presents the reasoning behind the idea of mainstreaming HIV/AIDS in existing development and humanitarian work, and Part 2 presents practical ideas for agencies that are seeking to mainstream HIV/AIDS into their work.

Part 1: The case for mainstreaming HIV/AIDS

Chapter 2 considers the two-way relationship between under-development and the causes and consequences of HIV/AIDS. It shows how the disease can make gender inequality worse, and claims that HIV/AIDS is a long-term development problem with no obvious solution.

Chapter 3 explores what mainstreaming means, by setting out the four main terms used in this book:

- *AIDS work*
- *integrated AIDS work*
- *external (programmatic) mainstreaming of AIDS*
- and *internal (organisational) mainstreaming of AIDS*.

It identifies similarities and differences between them, and gives practical examples of what the terms mean for development and humanitarian organisations.

Chapter 4 addresses the question 'Why mainstream HIV/AIDS?'. It considers some of the problems that may arise if development and humanitarian organisations fail to take AIDS into account in their ordinary work. It also responds to some objections to the idea of mainstreaming HIV/AIDS, and describes two problems which development organisations may meet when they do AIDS work.

Chapter 5 draws together all the elements of Part 1. It presents a 'web', showing four levels of influence on HIV transmission, and different kinds of response, both direct and indirect. Currently most of the global response to AIDS is direct; this chapter argues that all the influences need to be addressed and recommends that in AIDS-affected countries the indirect approach of mainstreaming should be the basic initial strategy for development and humanitarian agencies. Organisations with enough capacity, skills, and resources should ideally also engage in direct AIDS work; others might form partnerships with other agencies that are undertaking AIDS work.

Part 2: Ideas for mainstreaming HIV/AIDS

Chapter 6 provides some general strategies for initiating and sustaining mainstreaming, and proposes some guiding principles. Chapter 7 offers ideas for mainstreaming HIV/AIDS within the internal operations of development and humanitarian agencies, and Chapters 8 and 9 offer suggestions for external mainstreaming in development and humanitarian programmes respectively. Chapter 10 presents an overview of the issues and challenges involved in promoting and adopting the strategy of mainstreaming, and the book concludes with Chapter 11.

Using this book

If you are not sure about the basic facts of HIV/AIDS, you should first read Appendix I. It describes the ways in which HIV can be passed from one human to another, and the four stages through which someone who is infected with HIV passes: from initial infection to developing AIDS. The appendix also explains how patterns of HIV infection vary according to age, sex, ethnicity, wealth, and occupation.

You will find that most technical words or phrases are included in the book's glossary on pages ix–xii. Each of these words or phrases is shown in italics the first time that it is used in the main text.

Most readers will need to read Part 1 of the book before Part 2. However, if you are already convinced of the case for mainstreaming, you might read only Chapters 3 and 5 before going on to Part 2.

When you reach Part 2, you may want to prioritise reading Chapter 7, if you are particularly interested in ideas for mainstreaming HIV/AIDS within organisations; or Chapter 8, if you are mainly interested in development work; or Chapter 9, if your main concern is humanitarian work. Chapters 6 and 10 are relevant to all three types of mainstreaming.

Some of the ideas for mainstreaming in Part 2 are presented in more detail, with practical suggestions for implementation, in a series of Units published in *AIDS on the Agenda*. If you have access to the Internet, you may wish to download the Units, which are listed below, from http://www.oxfam.org.uk /what_we_do/issues/hivaids/aidsagenda.htm.

Unit 1	Researching the current internal impacts of AIDS
Unit 2	Predicting the internal impacts of AIDS
Unit 3	Assessing the impacts of AIDS education
Unit 4	Devising or adapting a workplace policy
Unit 5	Monitoring the internal impacts of AIDS and the effects of internal mainstreaming
Unit 6	Training for mainstreaming AIDS in development work
Unit 7	Undertaking community research for mainstreaming AIDS in development work
Unit 8	Adapting organisational systems
Unit 9	Training for mainstreaming AIDS in humanitarian work
Unit 10	Undertaking community research for mainstreaming AIDS in humanitarian work

2 | HIV/AIDS and under-development

Introduction

This chapter explores the two-way relationship between the causes and consequences of HIV/AIDS and factors of under-development. It examines how HIV/AIDS can make women's position in poor communities even more difficult than it already is, and argues that HIV/AIDS is a long-term problem of under-development for which there is no obvious solution. This fact points to the need for development and humanitarian agencies to address it through their on-going core programmes.

AIDS as a development issue

Since HIV was first identified at the beginning of the 1980s, HIV/AIDS has been understood and addressed in two main ways, which still predominate today. First, it has been treated as a purely medical problem, with a scientific focus on the biological effects of the virus, and developing ways to tackle it through medical interventions. Second, it has been treated as a behavioural problem which can be solved by individuals acting on information; the result is a focus on AIDS-education campaigns.

Although both of those approaches are essential – HIV/AIDS is both a medical and a behavioural issue – this book approaches the problem as one of development – or, more accurately, of under-development. AIDS has not affected all nations or all types of people equally. More than 90 per cent of HIV-positive people live in developing nations, and sub-Saharan Africa alone is thought to account for about two thirds of the global total of cases. The worst-affected region in the world, Southern Africa, is home to about two per cent of the world's population – but thirty per cent of all the people in the world who are living with HIV/AIDS live in Southern Africa. HIV flourishes where the conditions of under-development – poverty, disempowerment, gender inequality, and poor public services – make societies susceptible to HIV

BOX 1 Susceptibility and vulnerability

In this book, *susceptibility* refers to the likelihood of HIV infection. The cause of susceptibility may be biological: malnourished people who are in poor health are more likely to become infected with HIV, if exposed to it, than those who are well nourished and in better health. Susceptibility to HIV infection is also determined by much wider influences, such as culture, *livelihood* strategies, and the balance of power between men and women. For example, a woman living in a society where it is not acceptable for her to propose using a condom is, all other things being equal, more susceptible to HIV infection than a woman who lives in a society where women commonly carry and use condoms. The idea of susceptibility can apply to an individual or to groups of people. For example, one can consider if a particular organisation is likely, via its employees, to be more or less susceptible to HIV infections, or consider the probability of a society experiencing a severe HIV *epidemic*.

In this book the term *vulnerability* refers to the likelihood of HIV/AIDS having negative impacts. If a household is described as being vulnerable to the impacts of AIDS, this means that if one of its members is infected with HIV, that household is more likely to be harmed by the effects of AIDS than a household in more fortunate circumstances. For example, a household which has few assets and little support from family or friends, in a society which does not provide welfare support, is more vulnerable than a household with more wealth, supportive social structures, and access to assistance from the State. Again, the concept can be used on various scales, from the vulnerability of an individual or household, to the vulnerability of organisations or societies.

infection and undermine efforts to prevent its transmission. Furthermore, those same factors of under-development make societies vulnerable to the impacts of AIDS.

Figure 2.1 illustrates a model of the causes and consequences of HIV/ AIDS. On the **causes** side are the main factors which make individuals, groups, and whole populations more susceptible to HIV infection. In addition to these, other factors include labour migration, economic globalisation, and environmental damage. On the **consequences** side are some of the impacts of HIV infection and AIDS, as they affect households, communities, and nations. These effects are more severe where vulnerability to the impacts of AIDS is high; for example, where there are few means of support for individuals who fall sick and for families that become impoverished. The important thing to note is that the two sides of the model reinforce each other: high susceptibility leads to higher levels of HIV infection, which leads to AIDS; and where people are vulnerable to the impacts of AIDS, its consequences cause increased susceptibility, and so on.

Causes of susceptibility to HIV infection

We shall first consider the causes side of the model.

- **Poverty** can create susceptibility to HIV infection in many different ways.

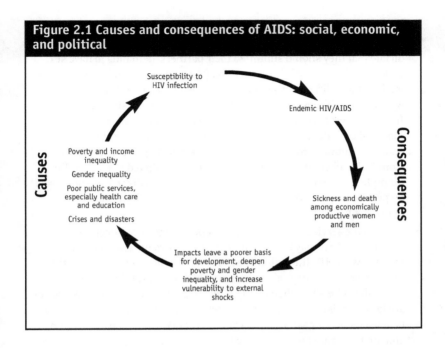

Figure 2.1 Causes and consequences of AIDS: social, economic, and political

Susceptibility to HIV infection

Endemic HIV/AIDS

Causes
Poverty and income inequality
Gender inequality
Poor public services, especially health care and education
Crises and disasters

Consequences

Sickness and death among economically productive women and men

Impacts leave a poorer basis for development, deepen poverty and gender inequality, and increase vulnerability to external shocks

In terms of biology, malnourishment and other infections weaken the body's *immune system*. Poverty also causes higher susceptibility to HIV infection because poor people are less able to afford health care, and so they are less likely to be in good health, less likely to get treatment for sexually transmitted infections (STIs), and less likely to buy and use condoms.

In general, poverty also has an important effect on how people think and act: it tends to displace long-term concerns such as the possibility of developing AIDS in the future. Poor people cannot afford to take long-term measures to protect their lives: they are too busy trying to survive in the short term. If they have few ways of earning a living, they may have to rely on selling sexual services; poor girls and women, in particular, may obtain cash, goods, protection, and favours, either via commercial sex work or through informal sexual exchange with varying degrees of commitment. When migrating to find work, young women may typically find themselves in employment which increases their susceptibility to HIV infection, such as working as house maids or bar girls. And men who migrate to find work are often separated from their homes and families for long periods, which may lead them to take casual sexual partners. Poor working conditions and living conditions can undermine people's health too, as experienced, for example, by the large numbers of migrant miners in Southern Africa.

- **Gender inequality** is another factor which increases susceptibility to HIV infection. Women and girls are made more susceptible if social norms dictate that they should submit to their partners' demands to have sex. Following the 'ABC' of HIV prevention ('Abstain, Be faithful, use Condoms') is all the more difficult in situations where women are likely to be punished with violence if they attempt to refuse sex or propose using condoms. In general, where girls and women have less control over their lives than men and boys do, and are disadvantaged in terms of education, income, and opportunities, they are less likely to be able to protect themselves from HIV infection. This susceptibility is partly linked to poverty; for example, where women's rights to inheritance and divorce are not respected, they are likely to become impoverished when widowed, or on leaving a relationship.

- **Poor public services** can increase susceptibility to HIV infection within a population. This may happen directly, when patients are accidentally infected with HIV through receiving contaminated blood in a transfusion, or when staff use surgical equipment which is not sterile or use unsterilised needles when giving injections. Such **modes of transmission** are far more likely in impoverished settings where blood for transfusions is not screened for safety, and health-care workers lack sterile equipment and are not trained in preventing the spread of HIV. Poor public services can increase susceptibility to HIV infection in indirect ways too. For example, where education services are inadequate and literacy rates, particularly among girls and women, are low, efforts to prevent infection are generally less effective, and there is greater inequality between men and women. And where treatment for STIs is not available, or not affordable, untreated infections leave those who suffer from them (and their sexual partners) more susceptible to HIV transmission.

- Finally, when considering the main causes of susceptibility to HIV infection, one must include the role of **crises** such as armed conflict or environmental disasters. In such situations the whole of the affected population may be more susceptible to infection with HIV as a result of impoverishment, displacement, loss of assets, and disruption to social-support networks. However, women and girls tend to suffer disproportionately, because they are more likely than men to be subject to rape and sexual violence, and they are more likely to resort to using their one portable asset – their bodies – in order that they and their dependants may survive. And where a crisis causes population movements, susceptibility may be further increased if populations with low levels of *HIV prevalence* encounter populations, or groups such as the armed forces, who are experiencing higher levels of prevalence.

Consequences of HIV infection

Until more research has been conducted into the consequences of HIV and AIDS, the impacts of AIDS are best understood at the levels of the individual and household. Analysts have identified sequences of reactions among AIDS-affected households in various settings; Table 2.1 illustrates a sequence of three phases.

How severe will the impacts of AIDS be? That depends on the level of vulnerability of the household and community. For each household, key factors which determine vulnerability include

- access to resources
- household size and composition
- access to assistance from extended families
- and the ability of the community to provide support.

Table 2.1 Household strategies in response to HIV/AIDS	
Phases	**Examples of strategies**
First Reversible strategies using *protective assets*	Seeking paid labour or migrating temporarily to find paid work
	Switching to the production of low-maintenance subsistence food crops (which are usually less nutritious)
	Taking money from savings accounts, or selling off stores of value such as jewellery or chicken or goats
	Getting help from extended family or community members
	Reducing consumption
	Borrowing from formal or informal sources of credit
	Reducing expenditure on non-essentials: education and non-urgent health care, for example
Second Strategies which are difficult to reverse, using *productive assets*	Selling land, equipment, tools, or animals used for farming or business
	Reducing the amount of land farmed and types of crop produced
	Borrowing at high interest rates
	Further reducing consumption and expenditure on education or health care
Third Destitution	Depending on charity
	Breaking up the household
	Migrating in desperation

(Source: adapted from Donahue (1998), which was adapted from M.A. Chen and E. Dunn (1996): *Household Economic Portfolios*, AIMS Paper, Harvard University and University of Missouri-Columbia – reprinted with the permission of the author.)

A household with enough resources in the form of labour, savings, and other assets will certainly feel the impact of a death from AIDS, but may be able to survive by using strategies from only the first stage of Table 2.1, and so recover from the shock. Poor households with fewer resources and fewer options are more vulnerable; they may reach the third stage, which is permanent impoverishment.

The vulnerability of households to the impacts of AIDS is also affected by the wider context, including the level of public services and support that is available from the State. In particular, people are less vulnerable where health care is available and is free or inexpensive, allowing HIV-positive people and their family members to get treatment even when AIDS is impoverishing them. This is all the more true where HIV-positive people have access to *antiretroviral therapies* which help them to live and work for longer. However, in the cycle of causes and consequences, the delivery of all services – from government, non-government organisations, and the private sector – may be affected by sickness and death among staff. Of particular note, as Chapter 4 will discuss, are the pressures that AIDS places on the health service, and the way in which a decline in education services can damage the prospects for future development. In addition, AIDS can threaten people's *food security*, and may make recovery from food shortages more difficult to achieve.

Two points are worth noting about the model of causes and consequences in Figure 2.1. First, the factors on the causes side are neither new nor special: poverty, gender inequality, poor public services, and crises created by armed conflict and environmental disaster were familiar issues long before HIV emerged. Any society with such problems is susceptible to HIV. But second, and in direct contrast, the consequences are both new and exceptional: AIDS affects economically productive people, with extreme negative effects in situations where people and societies are vulnerable to the impacts of AIDS. These are sufficient to reduce life expectancy dramatically and to reverse decades of development gains. Chapter 4 considers these impacts and their implications for development in more detail. The model suggests that the way to weaken the cycle of causes and consequences is through poverty-focused development work which, among many other benefits, makes the poorest people less susceptible to HIV infection and less vulnerable to the impacts of shocks such as AIDS.

Deepening gender inequality

It is clear that AIDS compounds poverty: when someone falls ill, the household loses that member's labour and income and those of the people who care for him or her; money is spent on treatment and perhaps also on false 'cures'; and the household pays for the cost of the burial. But it is less obvious that AIDS also deepens gender inequality. As gender issues are closely connected to HIV/AIDS, this section describes the ways in which AIDS has different consequences for men and women.

Consider a pair of twins, a sister and a brother who are both heterosexual. Even in a society where men and women are equal, the sister is biologically more susceptible to HIV infection than the brother, due to differences in their genitals and sexual fluids.[1]

If both the twins were to acquire a sexually transmitted infection, they would both be more likely to contract (and pass on) HIV. But the girl's STI is more likely to go untreated, because it is not as visible as her brother's. In addition, she may be less likely to seek treatment, because there is stronger social disapproval directed towards her for having contracted a sexually transmitted infection. Her brother's behaviour is more likely to be excused, or even approved of. And as an adult, the girl twin is more likely than her brother to have a blood transfusion, if complications arise during pregnancy and childbirth, and so she is more likely to acquire HIV from *unsafe medical procedures*.

If someone in the twins' household becomes ill with AIDS, the girl is more likely to be taken out of school before her brother – or not enrolled in the first place – in order to care for the affected person at home. Any pre-existing inequalities between the twins, including their working hours, access to education and health services, and nourishment levels, are likely to be made worse if the household is under stress.

Next, consider the twins' sexual partners. A pragmatic Nigerian proverb says 'No romance without finance' (Barnett and Whiteside 2002:85). Because sex is often connected to some form of exchange, it is probable that the girl's sexual partner or partners will be older than her, perhaps considerably so. Older men are more able than younger men to provide things for exchange: for example, money, practical goods, gifts such as clothes or beauty products, and social status. However, not only is the girl in a weak position in the relationship because she is a girl: the difference in age between her and her partner makes it even more difficult for her to influence sexual decision making, such as whether to use a condom or other form of contraception. Another problem for her is that older partners are also more likely to be infected with HIV than men of her own age, because they have been sexually active for longer.

In contrast to his twin sister, who is likely to find a sexual partner or partners easily and to get married before him, the boy may struggle to find a sexual partner or partners, because he lacks the attractions and resources of an older man. When he does have sex, however, he is in a position of greater power than his sister, regardless of the age of his partner or the nature of the relationship. He may well refuse to use a condom; but if he is determined to protect himself against infection, then he is able to do so.

Furthermore, if either twin is subjected to sexual abuse, forced sex, or rape, it is far more likely to be the girl than the boy. While it is true that boys and men are sexually abused and raped in many parts of the world, especially in prisons and the armed forces, the majority of abuse is directed at girls and women. This is true in the extreme circumstances of armed conflict, and also for the more ordinary *sexual and gender-based violence* which occurs within households and communities every day. Rough or violent sexual practices are more likely to cause injuries which increase the likelihood of HIV transmission.

If both twins were to become infected with HIV, it is probable that the sister would be infected first. If they lived in sub-Saharan Africa, for example, she would be two and a half times more likely than her brother to be infected between the ages of 15 and 24 (UNAIDS 2003:7). She would also, therefore, probably develop AIDS first. She might progress faster from infection with HIV to having AIDS, because she is more prone to being undernourished, and to having an immune system weakened by other health problems and the bodily demands of pregnancy and childbirth. However, while she would probably die before her brother – she in her twenties, he in his thirties – her sexual partner, being older, might well fall ill and die before her. She may have little control over the management of household resources, and she may find that their savings and capital are used up in her partner's search for effective treatment, leaving little money for her and her children's future. And, unlike her brother, she is likely to devote a lot of time to caring for her partner or other relatives when they are sick, because that is seen in her culture as women's work.

Finally, if the twins' partners die first, the impacts on them as widow and widower will also be unequal. Although details vary according to local custom, in general, the widowed brother would keep his property and maintain more control over his life – for example, deciding whether to take a new partner, and deciding who should care for his children. His sister is more likely to be dispossessed, to be sent back to her parental home, to be remarried by arrangement, and to have to care for the children without support from her partner's relatives. She may receive support from her brother, but she might also have to look after his children.

These are some of the ways in which the consequences of AIDS increase the basic inequality that is determined by gender. The situation is different, however, if the brother is having sex with other boys or men, and being penetrated by them. In that case he will be more biologically vulnerable than his sister, because HIV is transmitted through the anal passage more effectively than through the vagina. His social situation may be similar to hers if he is adopting a female gender role – if he is the subordinate partner with less control – and/or if he is having sex with older men in exchange for money or favours. However, he is likely to revert to male gender roles, adopting a position of relative power, if he also has sexual relationships with women.

A problem with no obvious solution

Agencies engaged in HIV/AIDS work sometimes speak of 'stopping HIV/AIDS'. But in the worst-affected regions of the world, HIV infection has become *endemic*, meaning that it is continuously prevalent and likely to be long-lasting. This book is based on the assumption that HIV/AIDS is here to stay, because there is no obvious solution to the problem.

Current medical treatment can extend the lives of HIV-positive people, and can reduce the numbers of babies who acquire HIV from their mothers, but it will be many years before there is a medical solution to the problem, such as an HIV vaccine, or a cure for AIDS. Even if a vaccine or cure were developed, it is unlikely that everyone would benefit. The majority of HIV-positive people in the world do not have access to basic drugs to treat *opportunistic infections*, let alone access to the latest antiretroviral therapies.

Focused behaviour-change programmes targeted at population sub-groups in specific locations can be effective; there has been success, for example, in projects which support gay men, injecting drug users, and brothel-based sex workers to protect themselves from HIV infection. However, given the current scale of the HIV *pandemic*, it is highly improbable that behaviour-change programmes alone can prevent all new infections. For that to happen, the 40 million people who are currently HIV-positive would need to live and die without passing HIV to anyone else. It is estimated that 90 per cent of them are unaware that they are infected with HIV.

Conclusion

> *There are no easy answers or simple technical and scientific solutions to dealing with the epidemic's spread and impact. The most effective response, or the best international 'vaccine' against this disease, is sustained, equitable development.*
> (Loewenson and Whiteside 2001:24)

This chapter has argued that HIV/AIDS is a problem of under-development and gender inequality, and furthermore that it is a long-term problem with no obvious solution. These two ways of seeing HIV/AIDS have important implications for how we think about responding to the pandemic.

First, the agreement that core development issues are of great significance to the spread of HIV and the impact of AIDS leads to the proposition that development work itself should be part of the response to the problem, in addition to direct AIDS work. Second, the argument that there is no immediate prospect of a resolution should divert attention away from short-term projects and simplistic 'solutions' – especially the idea that increased awareness leads to sufficient and sustained behaviour change to reduce the rate of HIV infection. Instead, seeing AIDS as an on-going problem suggests that attention to HIV/AIDS needs to be built into long-term development and humanitarian work.

This book argues that development and humanitarian agencies must face up to the long-term challenges of containing and coping with HIV infection and the impacts of AIDS, within their broader agenda of working for a fairer world. HIV/AIDS is not only an extraordinary issue to be addressed by scientists, activists, and specialists; it is also an everyday development issue, to be tackled by all development workers through their usual work. This book proposes that non-specialists should respond to HIV/AIDS indirectly, seeing it as a mainstream development issue which they can help to address through development and humanitarian work. The process by which non-specialists and non-specialist organisations can achieve this is the subject of this book: a process called 'mainstreaming'. The next chapter explains what mainstreaming means, with definitions and practical examples.

Note

1   A woman's genitals have a greater surface area of mucous membrane through which HIV can enter, and a young woman's risks are increased because of her immature cervix and thinner mucous membranes. Women's genitals 'hold' men's larger quantities of sexual fluids after intercourse, and the semen of HIV-positive men contains higher concentrations of the virus than the vaginal fluids of HIV-positive women. This is partly why, where HIV is predominantly transmitted through heterosexual sexual activity, more women are infected than men.

3 | What does 'mainstreaming' mean?

This chapter explains the main terms and meanings used in this book, and the distinctions between them, with definitions and examples.

The terms in brief

'*AIDS work*' is used to mean work which is directly focused on preventing HIV/AIDS, or care, treatment, or support for those who are infected – work which is **distinct, and implemented separately, from other existing development and humanitarian work.** For example, efforts to change people's behaviour, and home-based care programmes.

'*Integrated AIDS work*' is used to mean AIDS work which is implemented along with, or as part of, development and humanitarian work. The focus is still on direct prevention, care, treatment, or support, but with the difference that the work is **conducted in conjunction with, and linked to, other projects, or within wider programmes.** For example, HIV prevention as part of broader health-promotion programmes, or treatment as part of wider health services.

'*Mainstreaming HIV/AIDS externally*' refers to **adapting development and humanitarian programme work in order to take into account susceptibility to HIV transmission and vulnerability to the impacts of AIDS.** The focus is on core programme work in the changing context created by HIV/AIDS. For example, an agricultural project which is adjusted to the needs of vulnerable households in an AIDS-affected community.

'*Mainstreaming HIV/AIDS internally*' is about **changing organisational policy and practice in order to reduce the organisation's susceptibility to HIV infection and its vulnerability to the impacts of AIDS.** The focus is on HIV/AIDS and the organisation. It has two elements: direct AIDS work with staff, such as HIV prevention and treatment; and modifying the ways in which the organisation functions: for example, in terms of workforce planning and budgeting.

'*Complementary partnerships*' involve organisations focusing on their strengths, while **linking actively with other organisations that can address other aspects of the HIV/AIDS pandemic.** For example, an agricultural project forms a partnership with an *AIDS Support Organisation* (ASO). When agricultural extension workers are asked about HIV/AIDS by community members, or they encounter people needing home-based care, the workers are able to refer them to the ASO. Meanwhile, the agricultural project teaches the ASO's volunteers about the long-term impacts on livelihoods when AIDS-affected households sell off their assets in their search for a cure. As a result, the volunteers become more willing to discuss such matters with people who are living with HIV/AIDS and they thus help them to reduce the impacts of AIDS on the household. The ASO also refers vulnerable households among its clients to the agricultural project, which is able to provide support to those households which is relevant to their current and future needs.

Similarities and differences

The first two terms – *AIDS work* and *integrated AIDS work* – are the most similar, because they both refer to work which directly addresses AIDS through prevention and care. The precise line between AIDS work and integrated AIDS work may be difficult to locate, but the general types are easily recognised. Many AIDS projects, especially those of AIDS Support Organisations, are stand-alone interventions, while AIDS work undertaken within wider health and education programmes is comparatively integrated.

Internal mainstreaming includes *AIDS work* with staff, because an organisation's susceptibility to HIV infection and vulnerability to AIDS is largely determined by the level of HIV infection among its employees, and by their means of coping with AIDS. However, internal mainstreaming entails more than this, because the way in which the organisation functions also affects its susceptibility and vulnerability. By modifying how it operates with regard to internal issues such as recruitment, workforce planning, and budgeting strategies, an organisation can improve or protect the way in which it functions in a time of AIDS. This broader way of taking HIV/AIDS into account is shared with the strategy of *external mainstreaming*: rather than concentrating directly on AIDS, both forms of mainstreaming require a wider perspective of development work in a time of AIDS. Internal mainstreaming aims to ensure that organisations can continue to operate effectively, despite AIDS, while external mainstreaming is about ensuring that development and humanitarian work is relevant to the challenges presented by AIDS.

The biggest contrast among the terms is between *AIDS work*, whether stand-alone or integrated, and *external mainstreaming* of HIV/AIDS. While AIDS work focuses on goals related to AIDS, such as preventing HIV transmission, or improving care for people with AIDS, the focus of a project which has mainstreamed HIV/AIDS remains the original goal, for example improving *food security*, or raising literacy rates. Mainstreaming HIV/AIDS externally, as it is understood here, is not about initiating AIDS work. However, it is important to note that while AIDS work and external mainstreaming are different from each other, they both work against HIV/AIDS, and they complement each other. (See Appendix 2 for a graphic presentation of this point.)

Finally, the term *complementary partnerships* emphasises how AIDS work and development work can join together to tackle the problem. The notion behind complementary partnerships is that different types of organisation are better suited to undertaking different aspects of the response. Where possible, organisations should link together and benefit from each other's expertise; this is likely to be more effective than a situation in which each organisation tries separately to undertake all types of response.

Mainstreaming is not...

In addition to the definitions above, and the examples which follow, it may be useful to indicate a few ways of responding to HIV/AIDS which this book does not categorise as mainstreaming. For example, mainstreaming does not mean that other sectors take over the functions of the health sector. Also it is not concerned with completely changing an organisation's or sector's core functions and responsibilities, but instead it is concerned with viewing them from a different perspective, and making alterations as appropriate. Connected to this, mainstreaming is not about changing all work to serve only AIDS-affected people, nor necessarily ensuring that all projects are accessible to all people affected by AIDS.

How should a mainstreaming policy be implemented? It is not a single event, but a process. And internal mainstreaming involves more than doing AIDS work with staff, although that is important. Finally, mainstreaming is not about 'business as usual'; although some changes may be small, the process should result in changes which make the organisation better able to function in a context of AIDS, and make its work more relevant to that context.

Examples

The following examples aim to bring the terms to life, by describing the core functions of five organisations in five different development sectors, and suggesting what each might do if it were to adopt each of the five strategies listed at the start of this chapter. The examples are imaginary, but they are based on actual experiences.

Agricultural extension

Imagine that a CBO providing agricultural extension decides to respond to HIV/AIDS. Its core business is to help community members to improve their access to food and income. If the CBO were to begin a new AIDS project, recruiting and training Community AIDS Volunteers to promote and sell condoms, then it would be engaging in **AIDS work**. If instead it were to train its agricultural extension workers to promote and sell condoms to farmers, then the new AIDS work would be **integrated** with its existing work.

The CBO could, however, respond to the problem without doing any AIDS-focused work, by **mainstreaming HIV/AIDS externally**. Imagine that it does some research with households affected by AIDS and finds that it is excluding them from its programme: women are too busy caring for the sick to travel to farmer-training sessions, and adolescents (including orphans now in charge of their households) are too young to qualify for inclusion. The CBO responds by seeking out affected households that are keen to take part in the extension work and offers to organise training days on their land, so that members can attend and benefit from the labour input of the other trainees. The organisation also broadens its livestock programme to include rabbits and chickens, which are preferred by vulnerable families because they give quick returns and, as assets, are more divisible than cattle and goats.

The CBO is unsure how to work with young people, so it seeks advice from a youth-focused NGO operating in a nearby town. The two organisations realise that they can support each other, and they form a **complementary partnership**. The NGO provides training to the agricultural extension workers, challenging their prejudices against working with young people, and enabling their work to become more youth-friendly. The CBO provides agricultural expertise to the NGO, by running sessions about farming for the NGO's youth group.

As for **internal mainstreaming**, the CBO already has a policy on terminal diseases and provides medical and funeral benefits for staff members who are HIV-positive; but no one has considered how AIDS may affect the organisation in the future. A small team is formed and charged with predicting the likely impacts of AIDS on the organisation's finances and human resources, with a view to minimising those impacts. The team's work is limited by a lack of data, but its estimates suggest that within five years the costs will rise substantially, perhaps beyond the organisation's ability to pay. They establish management systems in order to gather accurate information on staff absenteeism, medical costs, and other benefits paid, and so they set in motion the process of reviewing the terminal-diseases policy. The strategy aims to ensure that the organisation can survive the financial impacts of AIDS.

Health promotion

A health-promotion agency sees its core business as increasing awareness and use of preventative and curative health measures; it does this mainly through the performance of community dramas. If it wanted to begin **AIDS work**, it might conduct AIDS education through a new programme of drama performances and video shows. If it preferred to do **integrated AIDS work**, it could fit messages about AIDS, sexual health, and *safer sex* into some of its other plays. But suppose the agency decides to **mainstream HIV/AIDS externally**. It begins by considering its existing work. It finds that its drama performances are popular because they create an entertaining community event, but that this, together with the presence of alcohol sellers, provides an environment for *unsafe sex*. Following consultation, the agency continues the drama work, but often performs to separate audiences of women, men, and young people. At evening performances for the whole community, the agency **integrates AIDS work** to reduce the likelihood of unsafe sex, by making sure that condoms and non-alcoholic drinks are available. The organisation also develops a new drama about alcohol use and unsafe sex, and uses it as a starting point for discussions with the audience. This leads to requests from community members for more information about HIV/AIDS and for personal support. As there are no local organisations offering counselling with whom the agency could form a **complementary partnership**, the managers decide to apply for funds to begin such a service.

The agency also begins work on **internal mainstreaming of HIV/AIDS**. It decides to address the long-tolerated problem that some of the staff who perform the dramas are engaging in unsafe sex with community members. It organises some discussion sessions on sexual health with male and female staff members in separate groups. Consultations with staff result in two new policies: a ban on alcohol consumption while working, and the facility to pay employees' field expenses into their bank accounts, rather than giving them cash. The agency also provides condoms for its employees, and, where possible, ensures that evening performances finish in time for the staff to return to their homes. Having begun discussing HIV/AIDS and their own potential for contracting and spreading infection, a few staff members press for a policy to increase staff awareness and provide health care.

Micro-finance services

Now take the case of an NGO providing micro-finance services through community groups. The staff see their core business as the provision of savings and credit schemes in order to support financially viable and productive activities. The NGO responds to the government's calls for all sectors to respond to the pandemic, and considers initiating a separate project of **AIDS work**, giving loans to people with AIDS, on terms and conditions different from those available to non-affected people in its core programme. However, by talking with other micro-finance institutions they learn that because repayment rates are likely to be low, this approach might not be sustainable. In any case, due to social stigma and low rates of HIV testing, it is unlikely that many people would apply for the loans. Instead, the NGO opts to **integrate AIDS work** with its existing work, by distributing leaflets about HIV prevention and AIDS to all the members of its micro-finance groups.

Later on, the NGO learns of **external mainstreaming**, and reviews its micro-finance work in order to understand how AIDS affects its clients and their participation in the micro-finance groups. It discovers several ways of modifying its approach in order to meet the needs of its clients when their households are affected by AIDS, without damaging the sustainability of the micro-finance groups or the NGO itself. These methods include allowing clients to miss meetings without penalties, and allowing them a 'rest' from the savings and credit cycle. The NGO also changes its rules so that other household members can take responsibility for the payment of loans, and can take on new loans, if the original member becomes sick or dies.

Although the NGO decides not to target loans to people with AIDS, it is able to form a **complementary partnership** with an AIDS Support Organisation which wants to begin an income-generating project with a group of HIV-positive people. The NGO is able to give advice on establishing appropriate rules and guidelines, and proposes two realistic aims for the project: that it should help the group members to avoid becoming completely impoverished, and encourage them to give each other moral support through working together. Meanwhile, the NGO provides funding to the ASO to visit each of its micro-finance groups to discuss HIV prevention and living with AIDS.

In the course of **internal mainstreaming**, the NGO discovers that it is over-reliant on two micro-finance specialists: if either or both became sick, the organisation's ability to do its work would be badly affected. It begins training and involving other staff in those functions, and standardising documentation systems so that everyone's work is more accessible and understandable to their colleagues. The NGO also talks to its donors to warn them about the possible future impacts on its capacity, if such key members of staff fall ill or die. One donor agrees to the NGO's proposal to add in extra budget lines to pay for temporary staff cover, and to plan for increased expenditure on recruitment and staff development.

Education

A Ministry of Education sees its core business as providing good-quality basic education for primary-school students. Engaging in **AIDS work** might involve supporting schools to set up anti-AIDS clubs, providing them with guidelines and basic promotional materials. **Integrated AIDS work** might consist of introducing topics of sexual health and HIV transmission into the school curriculum, or training school nurses in HIV prevention and basic counselling skills.

Mainstreaming HIV/AIDS externally would require research into the ministry's work, to learn how AIDS affects the demand for, and the quality and relevance of, education. For example, research with AIDS-affected households might reveal a variety of reasons why many girls and boys, including AIDS orphans, do not attend school, or do not attend regularly. The ministry might respond by providing scholarships or supporting expanded in-school feeding programmes, or by reducing school fees for children in need, including orphans. It could relax rules on compulsory school uniforms, or allow schools to operate more flexible timetables, in order to extend some education to those children who have to work during the day to support their families. Or it might put more emphasis on life-skills education, to equip pupils with practical skills which are relevant to their needs. In this regard, a **complementary partnership** might involve linking with the Ministry of Agriculture, to provide pupils with training in basic farming skills.

Internal mainstreaming would aim to reveal and deal with the threats that AIDS presents to the education system, and the ministry's ability to provide relevant services. If research shows that the supply of new teachers is less than the growing number lost to illness and death, the ministry might decide to invest in medical treatment for staff, to enable those who are HIV-positive to work for longer. It might also aim to increase the number of newly trained teachers. However, it learns that potential teachers, particularly women, find it difficult to attend the year-long residential teacher-training course. The ministry might respond to this constraint by introducing long-distance learning and in-service training. In the short term it could offer incentives to qualified teachers who have left the profession, to encourage them to return to teaching. The ministry might also begin an analysis of long-term implications for its workforce – not only teachers, but also members of the management, administration, and support functions.

Water and sanitation services

Finally, imagine a refugee camp where an NGO is responsible for water supply and sanitation. Its core business is to ensure that everyone has access to water which is fit for drinking, plus adequate washing facilities and latrines, so reducing illness caused by poor hygiene. The NGO is being encouraged by its main funder to respond to HIV/AIDS. It considers doing **AIDS work** through establishing a separate project, writing and distributing leaflets about HIV/AIDS, and promoting and distributing free condoms. However, it opts for an integrated approach, by starting to include HIV/AIDS and sexual-health education alongside its existing hygiene-education work.

The idea of **mainstreaming HIV/AIDS externally** is initially rejected by staff, because they do not see any connection between this problem and their water and sanitation work. However, an interested project officer begins to explore the possibility with users, and discovers two ways in which the NGO's work is linked to HIV and AIDS. First, many women are afraid to collect water, particularly after dark. Unbeknown to the NGO staff, there have been instances where women have been threatened and abused, including two who have been raped. The women would like lighting to be installed at the tap-stands, and for some taps to be moved to locations which they believe are safer. These measures would reduce their susceptibility to HIV infection, and improve their access to water. Second, the project officer's conversations with women reveal the out-of-sight needs of the people in the camp who are confined to bed, including those with AIDS. These people need a lot of water for washing, because of the fevers, vomiting, and diarrhoea from which they suffer. Carers cannot both look after them and collect adequate amounts of water; as a result, hygiene standards and infection control are getting worse. Carers would welcome the installation of tap-stands close at hand, assistance in collecting water, or special deliveries of water to bedridden people. The NGO discusses the problem with the agency responsible for health care in the camp, and they form a **complementary partnership** aimed at supporting carers in a variety of practical ways.

The NGO also starts work on **internal mainstreaming**, by examining its own functioning with regard to HIV transmission. It recognises that many of its staff are young, working and living away from home, and relatively wealthy and powerful, compared with the communities with whom they work. The NGO fears that some staff use their influence, or the organisation's resources, to buy sexual favours or to put pressure on refugees to supply sexual services. The NGO takes action by training all staff to understand how HIV is transmitted, and emphasises their responsibilities to the community members. The training also covers the disciplinary measures to be taken in cases of corruption and abuse, and a later incident provides the opportunity to demonstrate the commitment of managers to implementing the policies.

Summary

This chapter has defined and illustrated five strategies for responding to HIV/AIDS, which are summarised in Table 3.1. It is worth noting, however, that some activities may be hard to categorise, and that it could be argued that some types of work might belong to a different approach.

Table 3.1 Summary of terms, meanings, and examples

Term	Meaning	Focus	Examples
AIDS work	Interventions directly focused on HIV prevention and AIDS care	AIDS prevention, care, treatment, or support	Stand-alone behaviour change, treatment, or home-based care programmes
Integrated AIDS work	Interventions directly focused on HIV prevention and AIDS care	AIDS prevention, care, treatment, or support	Behaviour change, treatment, or home-based care programmes which are linked to, or part of, other work
Mainstreaming AIDS externally	Adapting development and humanitarian programme work to take into account susceptibility to HIV transmission and vulnerability to the impacts of AIDS	Core programme work in the context of changes related to AIDS	An agricultural project which is sensitive to the needs of vulnerable households in an AIDS-affected community
Mainstreaming AIDS internally	Changing organi-sational policy and practice in order to reduce the organi-sation's susceptibility to HIV infection and its vulnerability to the impacts of AIDS	AIDS and the organisation, now and in the future	AIDS work with staff, such as HIV prevention and treatment; and modifying how the organisation functions, for example, in terms of workforce planning, budgeting, and ways of working
Complementary partnerships	Organisations focusing on their strengths, and linking actively with other organisations that can address different aspects of the AIDS pandemic	Collaborating with those more able to address needs beyond the organisation's own expertise	An agricultural project and an AIDS Support Organisation linking to share their relative strengths and expertise

The examples in this chapter show that there is a lot of difference between AIDS work – whether it is separate or integrated – and mainstreaming HIV/AIDS externally. For the former, the starting point is the problem of AIDS, and AIDS projects are developed in response. For the latter, the starting point is organisations' existing development work, with processes modified as appropriate to take account of susceptibility to HIV transmission and vulnerability to the impacts of AIDS.

The term 'mainstreaming' is often used to refer to everyone doing AIDS work, or to AIDS work being present across budget lines; but this chapter has shown the distinct meaning given to the term in this book. In each of the five cases described above, the outcome of external mainstreaming is to adapt existing work in response to HIV/AIDS. In the cases of the health-promotion dramas and the sexual abuse linked to water collection, the adaptations aim to reduce people's susceptibility to HIV transmission. In the other examples, the modifications are concerned with reducing vulnerability to the impacts of AIDS. Each of those changes makes the existing work more relevant to those affected by AIDS, whether they are families needing agricultural advice, orphans wishing to attend school, members of micro-finance groups, or people confined to bed by AIDS.

This chapter has also shown that internal mainstreaming involves much more than organising seminars on HIV/AIDS for staff and ensuring supplies of condoms in the toilets. For the organisations engaged in health promotion and the provision of water and sanitation, mainstreaming raises the largely unacknowledged issue of unsafe sex and sexual bargaining between staff and community members. In the examples in this chapter, the micro-finance NGO and the Ministry of Education are both faced with human-resource issues which threaten the effectiveness of their work. And the agricultural CBO faces the task of balancing the rights and needs of staff infected with HIV against the organisation's survival.

Four of the examples include ways in which complementary partnerships might enable an organisation which is mainstreaming HIV/AIDS to link beneficially with others. However, it may often be the case, as with the example of the health-promotion agency, that there is no suitable organisation with which to link. The next two chapters set out the arguments for mainstreaming HIV/AIDS; they propose what different agencies might do in such a situation, depending on their capacity.

4 | Why mainstream HIV/AIDS?

Introduction

This chapter presents the arguments for mainstreaming HIV/AIDS both externally (in development and humanitarian programmes) and internally (within organisations). It responds to some objections to mainstreaming, and it also describes two challenges that are commonly faced by development organisations when they seek to integrate AIDS work into their programmes.

It should be noted that, owing to the limited experience of mainstreaming HIV/AIDS (in particular external mainstreaming) among development agencies, much of the argument is theoretical rather than being based on evidence.

The case for mainstreaming HIV/AIDS externally

Chapter 2 argued that HIV/AIDS is a development issue. Development work, in all its variety, ought to tackle both sides of the causes and consequences model shown in Figure 2.1. By, for example, reducing poverty, addressing inequality between men and women, and improving public services, development work should reduce both susceptibility to HIV infection and vulnerability to the impacts of AIDS. In an ideal world, this would occur without special effort: the development work would be totally participatory, and always sensitive to the variable needs, abilities, vulnerabilities, and options of different sections of the community. In the real world this is not the case. Without attending to HIV/AIDS through mainstreaming, development work may fail to exploit opportunities for reducing susceptibility to HIV infection, and for helping people to become less vulnerable to the impacts of AIDS.

Development work may even have negative effects, unintentionally increasing susceptibility and vulnerability. The possibility that development work could be working with, rather than against, AIDS – making things worse rather than better – seems unlikely, but it can happen, as this section will argue. It is important to note that the negative effects listed here are things which can and do happen, but this is not to say that development and humanitarian work always or even often has these unwanted effects, nor to devalue its positive impacts.

Development and humanitarian work may increase susceptibility to HIV infection

Effective development work undermines the causes of susceptibility to HIV infection, through processes of empowerment, poverty alleviation, raising the status of women, and improving public services. However, it can also, without intending to, increase susceptibility. For example, in rural communities, development workers may find it easy to attract sexual partners with their regular and relatively large income. Development workers may be more likely to engage in *unsafe sex* if they are based away from their families. In such situations, increased susceptibility to HIV infection applies to the development workers, their regular partners, and their other sexual partners from within the community. Sometimes the policies of the organisation may make things worse. For example, the Ministry of Education in Ghana has noted that its teachers often 'fall either in the category of those with high financial liquidity or the poorly resourced, as a result of the late reimbursement or payment of salaries. In the latter case the female teacher is at the mercy of those who can provide funds, and in the former especially the males become much "sought after" and have more bargaining power for sexual negotiations' (Ghana Ministry of Education 2002:x).

Furthermore, development workers may put pressure on community members to have sex with them. The scale of this abuse is unknown, but it is clear that individuals do sometimes use their position and their control over resources to exploit others. This may be particularly the case in emergency situations. A recent UNHCR investigation in West African refugee camps found evidence of a strong pattern of abuse against girls, mostly involving locally employed staff of international NGOs. More than 40 organisations were implicated in allegations that aid was refused unless paid for by sexual favours.

It is not only NGO staff who may use development resources to trade for sexual services, or to enable them to carry out sexual abuse: the possibility also extends to those community members who are given control over resources. For example, there is potential for abuse if the appointed caretakers in water projects are older men, while the water collectors are generally young women and girls. People can also acquire power through seizing control of development resources. In refugee camps, for example, self-appointed water monitors have used their control over scarce water supplies to pressurise women into providing sexual favours.

In setting up and running camps for refugees or displaced people, humanitarian agencies make decisions which indirectly affect people's susceptibility to HIV transmission. Some of the layout features known to enable sexual violence are communal latrines, and latrines and tap-stands located far away from dwellings, with inadequate lighting. Rapes may happen when girls and women have to leave the camp to gather firewood or water, and unaccompanied girls and women are sheltered unsuitably, for example on the edge of the camp. Distribution systems also encourage HIV transmission: if some people do not get their fair share, they may have to trade sexual favours in order to obtain food, clothing, and other essential items.

Unfortunately, successful development projects may also increase the likelihood of HIV transmission. For example, effective income-generating projects increase the amount of cash in households. This, it is assumed, is good, because the money will be spent on food, health care, and education. However, men may spend the additional money on alcohol and other recreational drugs, and on sex, through buying sexual services commercially or through maintaining relationships outside marriage. This is less likely to happen if women have control over the additional income. Similarly, improving access to markets allows people to get a better price for their products, but being away from home with an unusually large amount of money can lead men to take increased numbers of sexual partners, with a greater likelihood of unsafe sex. Where the additional income is controlled by men, susceptibility to HIV infection can be further increased if this leads to arguments within households, higher numbers of sexual partners, or divorce. In general, where development work focuses on increasing household income without regard to gender issues within the household, there is the danger that shifts in power in favour of men may increase susceptibility to HIV infection.

Finally, large-scale infrastructure projects have many unplanned effects on local people's lives, including their sexual health. The intrusion of moneyed and unaccompanied construction workers into an area is associated with rising STI rates. Significant improvements in transport infrastructure are also known to stimulate labour migration, leading to more families being separated for long periods of time, and an associated rise in numbers of sexual partners.

Of course, the implication of the problems raised here is not that development activities must stop, in order to avoid undesirable consequences. Rather, the point is to call attention to the potential negative implications of development and humanitarian efforts, which, through mainstreaming HIV/AIDS, agencies and communities may be able to avoid or at least reduce.

Development and humanitarian work may increase vulnerability to the impacts of AIDS

If development and humanitarian agencies always knew the changing needs in the communities whom they serve, and responded effectively to them, their work would automatically help households to cope with the consequences of AIDS. Development projects would benefit families who already had a member with AIDS, and not-yet-affected but vulnerable households which might, in the future, face similar problems. However, where agencies are not sensitive to the changes that AIDS is bringing, their work may make households more vulnerable to the impacts of AIDS, and so make its consequences worse.

In general, this may happen when the mode of development is poorly suited to the situation faced by people who are badly affected by AIDS. For example, an organisation may promote agricultural practices which require a lot of labour, or new methods of cultivation, harvesting, or processing which require the expenditure of cash. In some cases, agencies' ideas may make higher demands on labour and on cash, as in the case of labour-intensive cash crops requiring chemical fertiliser, or new methods of irrigation requiring high-maintenance channels and expenditure on pumps.

Without AIDS the new practices may be very successful: with enough labour and investment, the cash crops are profitable, and the irrigation produces much higher yields. Even in communities with high HIV prevalence, there are families who are not badly affected by AIDS, who may participate and benefit for some time. However, when AIDS strikes, there is the risk that what was beneficial becomes burdensome. The household can no longer meet the extra demands on labour; medical and funeral costs compete for cash with the new agricultural practices. Households which were initially suited to the new practices can no longer cope with them. Where land for food crops has been turned over to cash crops, or households have fallen into debt, they may be more vulnerable to the impacts of AIDS than if they had not adopted the new practices.

Development and humanitarian work may exclude households affected by AIDS

If development work is not sensitive to the consequences of AIDS and the varied needs of affected households, then it will often exclude them, without intending to, from the development process and its benefits. In the example given above, any household already directly experiencing AIDS would be unlikely to start cultivating cash crops, or adopting new irrigation methods. In addition to the shortage of labour or capital, there are social barriers (either perceived or real) to the members' participation, and they cannot spare the time needed to take part in the project. Exclusion may also occur in emergency situations where, for example, vulnerable people may not receive food rations because they cannot travel to distribution points, wait for distribution, and then carry the food home.

In general, members of AIDS-affected households, and particularly girls and women, are less likely to take advantage of development opportunities, such as literacy programmes and capacity-building exercises, or awareness-raising events. The usual reasons are lack of time and cash, but in some cases people may actually be made to withdraw from projects. In particular, micro-finance groups often require members to attend meetings regularly, and to repay their loans according to a schedule. These rules – which keep the groups together and oblige members to make payments on time – may mean that AIDS-affected members are excluded.

AIDS-affected people may also be excluded if development agencies fail to update their targeting strategies as household structures change. A focus on working with men as heads of households automatically excludes the increasing numbers of new, and highly vulnerable, forms of household in AIDS-affected communities: those comprising grandparents and orphans, or orphans living without adults, or female-headed households. Although the proportion of these vulnerable households may be significant, standard development work may ignore their needs. For example, a very small proportion of agricultural extension resources is directed at young farmers – not to mention children – and female farmers.

Exclusion is also likely to result where development staff have judgemental attitudes towards people affected by AIDS. In a recent survey of health professionals in Nigeria, one in five of the respondents stated that people who have HIV/AIDS have behaved immorally and deserve their fate. One in ten of the health workers said they had refused to care for someone whom they believed to be HIV-positive, or they had denied him or her admission to a hospital (UNAIDS 2003:31).

Problems may also arise if development professionals have negative ideas about the value of people with AIDS. If they are seen to be 'as good as dead', they will not be included in project activities, even during periods of improved health. This discrimination may extend to the sexual partners of people with AIDS, if others assume that they too are likely to be HIV-positive. A third element of discrimination arises from development workers' denial of, and distaste for, HIV/AIDS. If employees are trying to convince themselves that they are not at risk of HIV, or they wish to avoid meeting people who are visibly affected by AIDS, they will be biased against interacting with affected community members. In addition, where development agencies do not notice, or confront, discrimination against people with HIV/AIDS, their lack of action suggests that such behaviour is acceptable.

Finally, and significantly, AIDS-affected households are likely to be under-represented in consultations about community needs, and in community forums. Their members are also less likely to take on responsibilities through development structures such as village development committees. If they are not included at the needs-assessment stage of the project cycle, it is even more probable that they will be excluded at later stages.

AIDS contributes to failed development work

The previous three sections have shown how development work unfortunately may increase people's susceptibility to HIV transmission and their vulnerability to the impacts of AIDS. This is not to criticise the way in which development work changes things, but to note the potential for such work to produce unintended negative consequences in relation to HIV and AIDS. The rationale behind external mainstreaming of HIV/AIDS is that some of those adverse effects of programme work could be avoided. In addition, organisations could actively take advantage of opportunities to address susceptibility to HIV transmission and vulnerability to the impacts of AIDS indirectly through development work. There is, however, another strong argument for external mainstreaming: ignoring HIV/AIDS leads to failed development work. Even if that work does not have any of the negative effects described above, continuing with 'business as usual' in countries which are hard hit by AIDS means ineffective, or less effective, development work.

Capacity building and participation

If development objectives are to be met in the context of the HIV/AIDS pandemic, development agencies need to understand the ways in which it may undermine their efforts. Capacity building is a popular development strategy which is directly affected by AIDS. Where levels of HIV infection are high, it is inevitable that some of the trainees will develop AIDS, and their skills will be lost. In Malawi, for example, an FAO 'training of trainers' programme was threatened by the deaths of one in four of the trainers (Topouzis and du Guerny 1999:55). In situations where significant numbers of skilled staff are being lost to AIDS, it may be more realistic to plan training programmes aimed at capacity *maintenance*, rather than capacity *building*.

At the general level, as already argued, AIDS limits the participation of affected households, because labour is diverted to care for the sick and to the increased burden of everyday tasks. If agencies do not assess the needs of AIDS-affected households, and those households do not participate in the project activities, then the development process will certainly fail them. Moreover, AIDS can interfere with community-wide participation and the productivity of development staff, if frequent funerals and periods of mourning disrupt work.

Agriculture

In agriculture, the impacts of AIDS are linked to a combination of factors:

- reductions in the quality and quantity of labour
- loss of skills and experience
- and sales of productive assets.

Together, these impacts can contribute to food shortages, as experienced in Southern Africa in 2002–2003, where studies showed links between AIDS and the onset of household food insecurity.

The loss of labour is partly due to the fact that women spend less time on farming while they are caring for someone with AIDS; in an Ethiopian study, AIDS-affected households were found to be spending only two fifths of the time that non-affected families were devoting to agriculture (Loewenson and Whiteside 2001:10). Productive labour time may be lost to attendance at funerals and observing mourning customs. Where farming systems need certain tasks to be done at certain times, production may be particularly vulnerable to the effects of AIDS.

Most loss of labour, however, is due to deaths from AIDS. The FAO estimates that Uganda had, by the year 2000, already lost twelve per cent of its agricultural labour force to AIDS. By 2020, Namibia is forecast to lose one quarter of the people working in the agricultural sector (FAO 2001: Table 2). In East Africa, labour shortages have already produced many documented effects at the household level, including less land cultivated; delays in activities such as planting and weeding; more pests; loss of soil fertility; fewer crops per household; decline in livestock production; and lower yields. There have also been shifts from growing cash crops to crops for the household to eat, and from labour-intensive crops, such as bananas and beans, to less demanding – and often less nutritious – foods such as cassava and sweet potato (Topouzis 2001:4). A study found similar shifts in crops in Thailand, along with a reduction in the area under rice cultivation (Barnett and Whiteside 2002:231). Reduced yields and fewer crops are directly linked to deepening poverty and poorer nutrition. Furthermore, deaths among farmers are weakening the agricultural skills base: many are unable to pass their knowledge to their children before AIDS intervenes through illness and death.

The harsh consequences of AIDS for subsistence farming are also caused by diversion of cash to the treatment and burial of household members. Livelihood security is made more fragile when household resources are used to raise money for health care, funeral costs, or basic needs. This is particularly the case where productive resources such as equipment, land, or animals used in farming are sold off. A study in Thailand found that two fifths of affected households disposed of land after the death of an adult (Loewenson and Whiteside 2001:10). Some households have enough resources to withstand the costs of AIDS, and to maintain production by hiring labour; but for others the loss of labour and of productive assets causes a rapid and permanent fall in standard of living. All of these impacts on agriculture create a very difficult context for agricultural extension work, but it is clear that for projects to be successful, they need to take the impacts of AIDS into account. Where AIDS has a strong hold, projects that aim to increase overall production may be not be viable, and established working strategies may be irrelevant. For example, in sub-Saharan Africa, agricultural policies are generally based on the now questionable assumption that there is a plentiful supply of labour (Topouzis 2001:xii).

Health

With regard to health, the impacts of AIDS can be so great as to reverse the gains that have been made in key indicators, such as life expectancy at birth. For example, at the turn of the twenty-first century, life expectancy in Haiti was 49 years, whereas before AIDS it had been predicted to be 57 years. Without AIDS, Botswana was expected to have had a life expectancy of 71 years by 2001; instead, with AIDS, it was estimated to be 39 years (Barnett and Whiteside 2002:22). Furthermore, without widespread and effective access to antiretroviral therapies, life-expectancy rates will continue to fall, perhaps to as low as 30 years in some sub-Saharan nations.

AIDS is also affecting another key indicator: the under-five child-mortality rate. To take Zimbabwe as an example, in 2000 the child-mortality rate was three times higher than would have been expected without AIDS. About 70 per cent of deaths among children under the age of five were due to AIDS (Barnett and Whiteside 2002:23, 279).

It is obvious that AIDS has major impacts on health through its effects on people who are HIV-positive. In addition, however, AIDS also has various impacts on the health of the remaining population, the people who are not infected with HIV. One way is via the general impoverishment that AIDS brings to households and communities, leading to more work, poorer nutrition, and less access to health care. Another route is via other infectious diseases, primarily tuberculosis, which opportunistically infect HIV-positive people. Having HIV makes the development of active TB ten times more likely. If left untreated, each person with active TB infects, on average, ten to fifteen others, whether they are HIV-positive or not.

AIDS can also affect general standards of health care, as institutions try to respond to the increasing numbers of people who need treatment and care due to AIDS. For example, in Botswana, hospital admissions doubled in only six years, with at least half of all patients having an HIV-related condition. Overcrowding increases the probability that infections will be passed between patients, particularly where there is not enough space to isolate people with TB. Staffing is being affected not only by illness and death among health workers, but also because health professionals are escaping the stress by taking jobs in private practice, or in other countries (UNDP 2000:22). Clearly, for highly affected countries, the health sector faces many challenges, with AIDS directly affecting the health of the HIV-infected, indirectly affecting much of the rest of the population, and weakening service delivery. As with agriculture, the present and future impacts of AIDS may, without substantial increases in investment, make it impossible to improve general health standards.

Education

Education is generally regarded as a critical sector for the future development of a nation. This is all the more so in an era of AIDS, because education is charged with protecting the 'window of hope' – the uninfected children who are the next generation of workers and parents. Schools provide the opportunity to teach HIV-prevention messages; more significantly, education increases the potential for young people to use information to make choices and to plan for the future. Education also accelerates a range of socio-economic changes which reduce susceptibility to HIV infection through improving the skills of girls and of boys. Forecasts for highly affected countries, however, predict an environment in which maintaining education standards, let alone improving them, will prove challenging.

One impact of AIDS on the education sector is sickness and death among teachers and other professionals. In highly affected nations, governments must significantly increase the numbers of teachers that they are training, if they are to protect ratios of teachers to pupils. Another impact is that AIDS reduces the numbers of children who enrol and stay in school, and widens the gender gap between male and female enrolment. In some nations such as Brazil and Zimbabwe, where primary-school enrolment is high, rates are noticeably lower among orphans. In other countries such as Tanzania, where around two fifths of children do not attend school, orphans are part of a wider group of vulnerable children who do not have access to education.

The case for mainstreaming HIV/AIDS internally

As Chapter 3 explained, internal mainstreaming is concerned with reducing the impacts of AIDS on the ways in which organisations function, in an effort to maintain their effectiveness. In essence, the argument for mainstreaming is similar to the argument for taking out insurance: that organisations need to invest in the process in order to avoid or reduce inevitable future problems. The prospects for those organisations which do nothing are potentially very damaging.

Unfortunately, because few development organisations or government ministries monitor the indicators that AIDS affects, there is less evidence of the actual extent of the internal impacts of AIDS than one might expect. However, various types of impact are evident, and are presented in Table 4.1 under three headings:

- **direct costs**, referring to the money which the organisation must spend whenever there is a case of HIV/AIDS;

- **indirect costs**, referring to the loss of productivity that results from each case of HIV/AIDS, which means that the organisation can achieve less with the same workforce;

- **systemic costs**, referring to the ways in which the organisation suffers from the cumulative effects of impacts from multiple cases of HIV/AIDS.

Within any organisation, the series of effects begins with HIV infection among staff members and among their families. When HIV infection leads to AIDS-related illnesses, the organisation suffers from the periodic absence of the affected staff member, either because the employee is ill, or because the employee is caring for a sick relative. When an HIV-positive staff member becomes unable to work any more, the organisation loses skills, and the investments made in that person. On death, work stops so that colleagues can attend the funeral; several of the organisation's vehicles may be used to transport the coffin and mourners. Where there are medical and death-benefit insurance schemes, which may also cover employees' family members, the direct costs of treatment, final benefits, and burial costs must be met. Then there is the expense of advertising for, recruiting, and training a replacement member of staff.

All of these impacts multiply as more people are affected. Over time, absenteeism and the accelerated turnover of staff lead to lower productivity levels, and recruitment of suitably qualified replacements may become difficult. The unpredictable nature of absenteeism and death may severely strain the organisation's ways of working, while this and the experience of losing colleagues may harm staff morale and motivation. Finally, the costs of treatments and benefits, and of recruitment, may undermine investment in the organisation, or its work. In the extreme, they might threaten the financial viability of the organisation.

Internal mainstreaming cannot protect an organisation from all of these impacts – some are inevitable if a staff member develops AIDS – but it can reduce their severity. Internal mainstreaming aims to reduce susceptibility to HIV infection among staff members, and to help HIV-positive employees to manage their status through *positive living*. Establishing clear policies reduces the expense and stress incurred when managers have to make 'life or death' decisions about the welfare of their employees and their dependants. Internal mainstreaming also aims to modify organisational policies and systems to reduce the organisation's susceptibility and its vulnerability to the impacts of

Table 4.1 Workplace impacts of HIV and AIDS

DIRECT COSTS	INDIRECT COSTS	SYSTEMIC COSTS
Benefits package	**Absenteeism**	**Loss of workplace cohesion**
• Health care • Health insurance • Disability insurance • Pension fund • Death benefit • Funeral expenses	• Sick leave • Other leave (formal and informal) taken by sick employees • Compassionate leave • Attending funerals • Leave to care for dependants with AIDS	• Reduction in morale and motivation • Disruption of schedules and work teams • Breakdown of workplace discipline (unauthorised absences, theft)
Recruitment	**Sickness**	**Workforce quality**
• Costs of advertising and interviewing • Costs to productivity of vacant posts	• Reduced performance of individuals, due to HIV/AIDS sickness while working	• Reduction in average levels of skill, performance, institutional memory, and experience of employees
Training	**Management resources**	**Quality of employment**
• Induction • In-service and on-the-job training costs	• Managers' time and effort responding to workplace impacts	• Cumulative costs reduce the quality of the workplace environment and reputation of the organisation

Source: adapted from Barnett and Whiteside 2002:256, and reproduced with the permission of the publisher, Palgrave Macmillan

AIDS through absenteeism and higher levels of staff turnover. Finally, internal mainstreaming involves doing research to predict, and protect the organisation from, any financial problems which may be caused by AIDS. These strategies are considered in more detail in Chapter 7.

In addition to the direct benefits for organisations which mainstream HIV/AIDS internally, there may also be some advantages for organisations which mainstream when others do not. An agency which has strong and supportive HIV policies and whose managers are coping with the challenges that AIDS presents is likely to be a more attractive place to work, and better able to recruit and retain qualified staff. And if its work is relatively effective despite AIDS, compared with organisations struggling with absenteeism, vacant posts, and low morale, the agency may be better able to attract funding and use it to good effect. Significantly, the organisation which has successfully mainstreamed internally is likely also to have a greater ability to respond to HIV/AIDS in its programme work, whether through external mainstreaming or AIDS work, because its staff should better accept and understand the condition in all its complexity, and because they and the organisation will be more likely to practise what they preach.

While it is argued here that internal mainstreaming of HIV/AIDS makes sense for all organisations, particularly in highly affected countries, it is likely to be more challenging for small organisations, due to a combination of two factors. First, for an organisation with a small number of employees, it is hard to predict if and when AIDS may have an impact. Even where HIV prevalence is high, such an organisation might enjoy many years without any employees falling ill. Conversely, it might lose a significant proportion of its workforce in a single year. Second, small organisations typically have fewer resources on which to draw, and so are more vulnerable to the impacts of AIDS, such as loss of workers to absenteeism and increased health-care and funeral costs. The situation for many small organisations is similar to that of poor households: those with poor resources are most vulnerable to AIDS, and most likely to be badly affected by it.

Arguments against mainstreaming HIV/AIDS

Having reviewed the rationale for mainstreaming, this section addresses some possible objections to the idea.

'Mainstreaming is a distraction'

Mainstreaming may be seen as a threat by those agencies that believe that 'we must all act now to fight AIDS', because it proposes a strategy which might divert resources away from doing direct AIDS work. Where there is a need for more agencies to get involved in AIDS work – for example, where a population lacks basic information about HIV and AIDS, or where HIV-testing facilities are not available – then the notion of mainstreaming may seem like a distraction, or a low priority. Mainstreaming also seems to ignore what appear to be the obvious issues requiring attention: HIV transmission, illness, and death. However, the notion that all agencies should prioritise AIDS work is problematic, for two main reasons.

First, development organisations are not all equally suited to undertaking AIDS work. Some are well suited to it, by virtue of their capacity, experience, relationships with particular groups within the community, and involvement of people directly affected by AIDS. Others are in a comparatively weak position: for example, they are small in size, have no experience in sexual-health issues, work in unrelated fields, or lack the capacity to take on new and unfamiliar work. They are probably better placed to mainstream HIV/AIDS in their existing work. It is important to recognise that poor-quality AIDS work can be ineffective and thus waste limited funds. It may also be damaging: for instance, if it seems to put blame upon 'high-risk' people, or people with AIDS, or if it impoverishes the beneficiaries of income-generating activities that are not viable. Common mistakes in AIDS work can also undermine other agencies' efforts: for example, through unsustainable welfare programmes, or loans made with little expectation of repayment. The additional workload involved in taking on AIDS work can also harm an organisation's core work. In particular, where the decision to respond to AIDS is funding-led, an organisation's former projects and target groups may easily become neglected.

Second, the many problems of underdevelopment persist, and, as Chapter 2 argued, they are allowing the pandemic to flourish. Hence, core development work is needed more than ever. If HIV/AIDS is mainstreamed in it, such development work can also tackle the causes of HIV susceptibility, and help to reduce vulnerability to the impacts of AIDS. But failing to mainstream can lead to the various problems described at the beginning of this chapter – making people more susceptible, or more vulnerable, excluding people from development, and making development organisations ineffectual – all of which lead to ineffective development work. If that analysis is true, then mainstreaming HIV/AIDS is crucial for responding to the pandemic, and for ensuring that development work and AIDS work are working together against AIDS. In this sense, mainstreaming is not a distraction but a critical, additional strategy.

'Mainstreaming is an excuse to do nothing'

One of the concerns about mainstreaming gender, which also applies to HIV/AIDS, is that the process makes it difficult to see what the organisation is doing about the issue – whether gender inequality or AIDS. It is very obvious if an organisation has special women's projects, or focused AIDS work, but it is not immediately apparent whether concerns about gender or AIDS are being addressed within general development and humanitarian programmes. This leads to the suspicion that an organisation can use mainstreaming as an excuse for not acting directly, but can claim to have addressed the issue without having done very much.

It is a question of credibility and honesty. Organisations which tend to exaggerate their achievements can also do so if undertaking direct AIDS work – for example, claiming to run comprehensive prevention programmes, but actually doing little more than delivering lectures and distributing leaflets. It would not be fair to reject the idea of mainstreaming on the basis that it may be used cynically: any development strategy is open to misuse, particularly if it can attract funding.

In any case, mainstreaming HIV/AIDS is not an easy option. As Part 2 of the book will show, it is a fairly complex and on-going process which requires the involvement and commitment of people throughout an organisation. Far from being an excuse to do nothing, mainstreaming means reflecting, assessing, making connections, and acting on both internal and external issues. Systems for institutionalising and monitoring the process can ensure that HIV/AIDS is not mainstreamed into non-existence, but is rather a permanent concern which is present within all development and humanitarian work.

'Mainstreaming is unnecessary'

Development practitioners who are already listening to the concerns of community members, for example through participatory appraisals, may feel that they do not need a special mainstreaming strategy for HIV/AIDS. They would expect AIDS-related issues to arise from their needs assessments, and to be dealt with through the normal project cycle. Someone who read a draft copy of this book wrote in the margin: '*Is this very different from what we should be doing anyway?*' In many ways she is right. However, there are several reasons why the work of development and humanitarian agencies may not achieve the results that mainstreaming proposes.

Many of the constraints stem from staff skills and attitudes. Workers who refuse to believe in HIV/AIDS, who understand it as a product of witchcraft or punishment for immoral behaviour, or who are fearful of people with AIDS, will not be able to tackle the problem constructively at community level. Internal mainstreaming is partly about helping staff members to address their own fears, prejudices, and denial, so that they can better understand the condition as it affects them and others. Staff are also likely to need training in order to assess needs among various groups within the community, because issues relating to AIDS – including death, sex, sexual health, and sexual violence – are sensitive topics which are unlikely to emerge unless staff ask the right questions in the right way. Furthermore, without training to understand the complexity of HIV/AIDS, development workers may miss the relevance of apparently unconnected issues, such as the significance of who in the household receives the profits of income-generating activities. Untrained staff are also likely to be unaware of the possibility that their work might need to be modified: for example, if it is excluding some households or groups of people.

Another problem is that the issues faced by AIDS-affected households may not emerge during project appraisals. Participants who are directly affected by AIDS may not speak up, fearing the stigma which revelation may bring. And, as this chapter has already stated, those individuals who are most susceptible and vulnerable may be unable to spare the time to take part in assessment exercises. While large numbers of organisations use participatory appraisal techniques, such methods, unless used thoroughly, may not lead to rigorous analysis of vulnerability, or of ways in which people are socially excluded, or of differences within communities and within households. External mainstreaming involves deliberately seeking the input of affected households. Moreover, 'affected households' are not all the same: development workers need to learn about the differing needs of people in differing situations, such as those who are ill, recovered, widowed, orphaned, or newly heading a household.

Other constraints, which could be dealt with through internal mainstreaming, stem from organisational systems. If an organisation plans only a few years ahead, it may lack the long-term perspective that is needed to consider, and act upon, the future impacts of AIDS. If funding is closely linked to specific sectors, and AIDS is seen as a health issue, then 'unrelated' activities, such as agriculture, may not qualify for funds for AIDS-related expenditure. If job descriptions and terms of reference do not routinely include attention to HIV/AIDS, then staff and consultants may forget or deny their responsibility for taking it into account. And if an organisation's personnel procedures lack confidentiality and do not support HIV-positive staff, a culture of denial and discrimination may prevail, leaving it poorly placed to consider and respond to AIDS internally or externally. Thus, not only is external mainstreaming necessary to ensure that HIV/AIDS and the needs of AIDS-affected households are taken into account in programme work, but internal mainstreaming is needed to enable organisations to respond indirectly but fully to HIV and AIDS.

'Mainstreaming is not feasible in an emergency'

The idea of mainstreaming HIV/AIDS will be resisted by those working in humanitarian programmes, if they consider the additional demands to be unrealistic and unnecessary. However, although some aspects of mainstreaming HIV/AIDS involve additional work, many of the relevant measures already form part of the good practice to which humanitarian organisations aspire. To a large extent, then, if such good practice is realistic – through better preparedness, training, funding, planning, and implementation – then so too is the proposal to mainstream. For example, in refugee camps it is routinely accepted that agencies should listen to and involve residents, and particularly women and young people, in planning the layout and main functions of the camp. The same listening and involvement are crucial mechanisms for mainstreaming HIV/AIDS. Positioning toilets, tap-stands, and lighting in ways that discourage sexual violence is a basic aspect of protection in refugee camps, and these precautions also reduce susceptibility to HIV transmission associated with forced sex and rape. Treatment for STIs is part of the recommended health-care package once an emergency situation has stabilised, and it also helps to reduce HIV transmission. And in food-aid distributions, agencies aim to ensure that the most vulnerable people receive their rations, which should include those affected by chronic illness, including AIDS.

Moreover, while responding to HIV/AIDS indirectly may appear to be unnecessary, emergency situations, and particularly those involving conflict, create virtually all the conditions that are likely to increase susceptibility to and transmission of HIV. The future effects of not responding are higher levels of HIV infection, and the many interconnected ways in which AIDS undermines reconstruction and development. Failing to mainstream HIV/AIDS in emergency programmes could have damaging effects during the crisis – for example, through sexual violence – and for generations afterwards through the impacts of HIV infection.

'Mainstreaming is irrelevant where HIV rates are low'

There seem to be three possible strategies to adopt with regard to main-streaming in situations where HIV prevalence is low, or where the impacts of AIDS are not yet evident. The first is to do nothing. The second is to encourage mainstreaming of HIV/AIDS anyway, but at a lower level of intensity than in a high-prevalence setting. This strategy involves engaging in the same processes of mainstreaming externally and internally, with the advantage that organisations would be well prepared when, or if, HIV rates begin to rise. The disadvantage is that it is very hard to motivate people to respond in advance if they see AIDS as a distant threat whose impacts are as yet generally invisible.

The third strategy is to focus on mainstreaming gender-related concerns, because these are ever-present issues which are important for development, regardless of HIV/AIDS. In programme work, external mainstreaming of gender equality might lead to adaptations to empower women; to reduce sexual violence; and to modify work in order to help impoverished female-headed households to improve their food security and become less vulnerable to external shocks. Such efforts can tackle immediate problems, while also addressing factors linked to HIV susceptibility and vulnerability to the impacts of AIDS. Meanwhile, internal mainstreaming of gender equality would help staff members to understand and act upon the links between their work and problems of gender, and would reduce gender-based discrimination within organisations. Internal mainstreaming could also involve measures such as developing a policy on responding to chronic or long-term illness (to include AIDS); putting in place policies to prevent discrimination in employment (including discrimination according to

HIV status); and improving systems such as ways of covering for staff absences.

The third strategy of mainstreaming gender equity does not, however, mean that mainstreaming HIV/AIDS would be unnecessary if infection rates subsequently rose. Although mainstreaming HIV/AIDS would probably be facilitated by the earlier work on gender, work to understand the impacts of AIDS at the household level and to learn from AIDS-affected households would still be needed. Much of the process of internal mainstreaming of HIV/AIDS would also need to be addressed.

Of course, as this book argues throughout, in the overall response to the problem, the strategy of mainstreaming is additional to that of direct AIDS work. In situations where HIV prevalence is low because HIV infection is concentrated among sub-groups of the population, development agencies with suitable experience and capacity may well focus on undertaking AIDS work with such groups: for example, working with injecting drug users or commercial sex workers, both to help them personally and to help to prevent HIV from crossing over into the general population.

Problems faced by development agencies undertaking AIDS work

This section presents two challenges specific to integrating AIDS work, and describes how they relate to the agenda for mainstreaming HIV/AIDS.

AIDS work may not be the community's priority

A recurrent problem for agencies implementing AIDS work is that fighting poverty and other issues are the stated priorities of community members, rather than AIDS. While this may be partly due to stigma and lack of awareness of HIV and AIDS, it could also be linked to the urgent nature of other problems confronting people.

One option is to meet people's priority needs first. In most cases, however, organisations intending to do AIDS work are unable to respond first to diverse needs such as food security or access to clean water or schooling, because they lack the time, funding, remit, and skills to do so. Instead, they may decide to proceed with an AIDS agenda, with or without engaging community members.

With mainstreaming, however, the question of whether or not HIV/AIDS is a community priority does not apply, because the aim is not to implement direct AIDS work, but to modify existing work as necessary. Mainstreaming, then, avoids the danger of imposing AIDS work, because it is about addressing HIV/AIDS indirectly, through development and humanitarian work which – ideally – does reflect communities' priorities. This might enable organisations doing AIDS work to make more impact by engaging community members in a wider response to the problem.

AIDS work is not the responsibility of every profession

Addressing HIV/AIDS as a development issue is often understood as requiring all sectors, and all development workers, to take on responsibility for responding directly to HIV and AIDS. This is most commonly expressed, and implemented, by field workers who are not health specialists taking on the role of HIV/AIDS educators. However, sectors and individuals in them often fail to accept and act upon the idea. This may be partly because they are not convinced that such work is their responsibility, and partly due to a lack of confidence in their own ability to do the work, or to distaste for having to discuss sexual issues. A further constraint is lack of time, given that AIDS work is almost always added on top of existing work commitments, which may affect morale and cause resentment among overworked staff. All of this points to two likely effects: that the AIDS work may not be of good quality, and that the increased workload may have negative impacts on the quality of core development work.

Although mainstreaming still requires time and energy, it does not demand that all development workers must be convinced that AIDS work is their responsibility, nor that they must take on new work. Instead, they must bring HIV/AIDS into focus as another important influence on the lives and prospects of the people with whom they work, and consider if they need to make any changes to the way in which they work in the light of the changes brought about by the pandemic.

Summary

This chapter has described three ways in which development and humanitarian work may unwittingly work with, rather than against, AIDS: increasing susceptibility to HIV infection; increasing vulnerability to the impacts of AIDS; and excluding those affected by AIDS from the development process. This chapter has also reviewed the ways in which AIDS can cause development work to fail, and how it can undermine the very functioning and sustainability of development organisations and other institutions.

The chapter then responded to five arguments against mainstreaming HIV/AIDS, and, described two problems with the strategy of integrating AIDS work in development work which are not encountered when mainstreaming. Overall, the chapter has aimed to explain the reasoning behind the idea of mainstreaming. The next chapter considers the implications for development and humanitarian agencies in terms of their response to HIV/AIDS.

5 | Implications for responding to HIV/AIDS

So far, this book has presented some of the thinking behind mainstreaming HIV/AIDS, and has given definitions and examples of mainstreaming and AIDS work. But what does the argument for mainstreaming mean in actual practice? How might development and humanitarian agencies best respond to the pandemic?

Adding mainstreaming to the menu of responses

Currently, the dominant response to AIDS is direct AIDS work, whether stand-alone or integrated. This is clear from the examples of the different terms and their meanings given in Chapter 3: the illustrations of AIDS work are easily related to actual projects, while those of mainstreaming are unfamiliar, and far from being common practice.

In general, direct AIDS work is seen to be the only possible response to the pandemic. An organisation seeking to address the problem feels that it must select from the menu of existing AIDS-work initiatives, including education, condom promotion, STI treatment, voluntary counselling and testing, treatment and care, support for HIV-positive people, and orphan support. This is partly because the idea of mainstreaming is underdeveloped, and there is little experience so far for agencies to learn from and copy. It is also because there is a very strong feeling among people responding to the pandemic that they should do direct AIDS work; in particular, there is a desire to inform and educate others, in order to help them to protect themselves against HIV infection.

The response of initiating AIDS work, regardless of the existing work of the organisation, is most evident in the way in which HIV education is added on to other development work. In some cases, this may be very straightforward. For example, in Malawi, the Ministry of Agriculture has sometimes included leaflets about AIDS inside packets of seeds. This is a low-cost means of spreading basic information, though arguably not very effective if done in isolation from other efforts. A more expensive strategy is to invest in training agricultural extension workers to conduct AIDS education. However, limited feedback suggests that few extension workers discuss AIDS or give out condoms, because they are too embarrassed, and they believe that it is a matter for specialist health workers. Where extension staff do engage in AIDS education, there is little evidence that their efforts lead to behaviour change, while they spend less time doing their much-needed agricultural development work.

This example illustrates two problems that arise if AIDS work is seen to be the only way of responding to AIDS. As already mentioned in Chapter 4, some organisations and their staff are not well suited to doing AIDS work; for example, if they have no experience in behaviour-change work or community-based approaches. As a result, their AIDS work may be ineffective or even damaging, for example if they communicate HIV-prevention messages which stigmatise sex workers. And taking on additional AIDS work may cause their core work to suffer if they do not have enough capacity to do both. Other organisations which are not well suited to doing AIDS work may opt to do nothing. In either case – whether organisations do or do not take on AIDS work – they fail to consider the basic strategy of responding indirectly through mainstreaming, because that option does not appear on the current menu of 'responses to HIV/AIDS'. The outcome is that an organisation's core work fails to address the problem – a fact which, as the previous chapter argued, can be harmful or, at best, a missed opportunity to improve its indirect contribution to the wider response to HIV/AIDS.

Direct and indirect responses

This book proposes that both direct and indirect responses to HIV/AIDS are needed, in order to address the wide range of factors which influence the spread of HIV and the impacts of AIDS.

There are many different reasons behind the spread of diseases. Figure 5.1 illustrates the factors influencing the HIV/AIDS pandemic, with HIV at the centre of a spider's web, and the factors that encourage the spread of infection and compound the impacts of AIDS spiralling outwards. Nearest to the centre of the web are the **bio-medical factors** which influence the likelihood of HIV transmission, such as different types of HIV, and the susceptibility of the individual according to his or her state of health (including the presence of STIs). Beyond those medical factors lie the **behavioural factors**, such as the number of sexual partners, the age gap between them, and use of condoms. The web then spirals further out to the **micro-environment** in which people live, including social, cultural, and economic influences which affect their

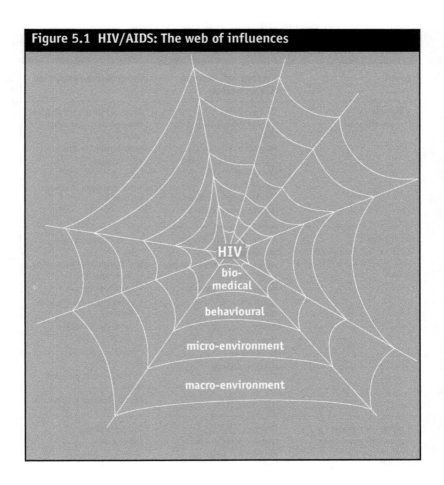

Figure 5.1 HIV/AIDS: The web of influences

HIV
bio-medical
behavioural
micro-environment
macro-environment

decision making and sexual behaviour, such as gender relations, poverty, and migration. The outside edges of the web concern the **macro-environment** of regional, and finally global, factors, including national wealth, income distribution, and the effects of conflict.

Table 5.1 presents the web's categories, together with a list (not complete) of factors that influence why people become infected with HIV, together with relevant programme responses. The programme responses under levels 1 and 2 relate mainly to direct forms of AIDS work, while those for levels 3 and 4 are indirect ways of tackling AIDS along with wider development problems. Clearly, each level is suited to particular professions and types of organisation.

Table 5.1 Factors influencing HIV infection, and programme responses to it

Level	Factors influencing HIV infection	Programme responses
1 Bio-medical *Focus on the body*	Virus sub-types Stage of infection and viral load Presence of STIs Physiology – women more susceptible Circumcision Unsafe medical procedures Immune-system status	Research into vaccine and cure Treatment of opportunistic infections Antiretroviral treatment STI treatment Condoms Blood screening, sterilising equipment
2 Behavioural *Focus on what men, women, boys, and girls do, or have done to them*	Number of sexual partners Rate of partner change Having several partners at the same time Age gap between partners Sexual practices Condom use Violent sex Rape Alcohol use Injecting drug use	Provide information and education Seek sexual-behaviour change: • fewer partners • use of condoms • delay beginning of sexual activity • same-age partners • get STIs treated Promote and distribute condoms Voluntary counselling and testing Needle-exchange programmes
3 Micro-environment *Focus on the local context in which men, women, boys, and girls live*	Poverty Women's rights and status Health status and access to health care Literacy Mobility and migration Levels of violence Gender norms, cultural practices and traditions	Poverty reduction Empowerment Nutrition programmes Health care Education Livelihoods security Promotion of human rights Legal reform
4 Macro-environment *Focus on national and global contexts*	National wealth Income distribution Governance International trade Natural disasters and climate change Conflict	Economic policy Taxation Redistributive social policy Good governance Terms of trade Debt relief Promotion of human rights

(Source: adapted from Barnett and Whiteside (2002:78), and reproduced with the permission of Palgrave Macmillan)

The first level, **bio-medicine**, is plainly the domain of medical scientists, health professionals, and traditional healers. This is where many organisations which deliver health services, including governments, NGOs, ASOs, and faith-based agencies, are most likely to operate, offering direct AIDS work through treatment and care.

The second level, relating to **behaviour**, is probably best addressed by local individuals and indigenous CBOs, such as community leaders, ASOs, and faith-based organisations, as well as the health sector, offering AIDS work in the form of HIV-prevention programmes and counselling.

The third level, that of the **micro-environment**, is mainly the realm of local government and development and humanitarian NGOs, undertaking indirect AIDS work by acting on the local development-related causes and consequences of AIDS.

And finally, the fourth level, the **macro-environment**, is the mandate of the State and international agencies such as the United Nations and World Trade Organisation, and the organisations which aim to influence them through advocacy, acting indirectly on the global issues which help to fuel the pandemic.

Implications for development and humanitarian agencies

If, as this book has argued, HIV/AIDS is a long-term problem of under-development which cannot be solved by working at levels 1 and 2, then action at all four levels of the spider's web is needed. This should lead to a better overall response to HIV/AIDS, involving all sectors and comprising both direct and indirect approaches. Furthermore, the combined effects of the work of organisations across sectors in responding to the pandemic are likely to be greatest if each agency begins by focusing on what it does best. This leads to the following implications:

- **Internal issues:** all organisations employ staff who may be or may become HIV-positive. As such, all organisations are vulnerable, to some extent, to the impacts of AIDS. This implies that they all need to engage with the strategy of mainstreaming HIV/AIDS internally, if they are to function effectively into the future. This applies to organisations operating at all levels of the spider's web, from small ASOs to international NGOs and government ministries. In settings of low HIV prevalence, certain elements of internal mainstreaming are likely to be fruitful, as Chapter 10 will explain.

- **Programme issues:** for organisations engaged in medical and behavioural AIDS work at levels 1 and 2 of the web, external mainstreaming may be useful. However, because those organisations should already be focused on and directly engaged with the issues raised by AIDS, mainstreaming is likely to be less relevant to them. After all, the meaning given to mainstreaming in this book is the modification of development and humanitarian work, in order to take HIV/AIDS into account and to act indirectly upon it.

- Development and humanitarian organisations generally engage in work at the third level of the spider's web, and they all work with people who are susceptible and vulnerable, to some extent. To ensure that their existing programme work is indirectly working *against* rather than *with* AIDS – that it is helping to minimise susceptibility to HIV transmission and vulnerability to the impacts of AIDS, rather than making them worse – all those organisations need to mainstream HIV/AIDS externally. Similarly, those agencies operating on the macro-issues at the fourth level of the web need to ensure that they mainstream HIV/AIDS, so that their policies take account of HIV transmission and the impacts of AIDS. As was argued in Chapter 4, in low-prevalence situations it may make sense to engage in a scaled-down process of external mainstreaming, or a similar process focused on related and immediate issues such as gender equality.

This book, then, proposes that internal mainstreaming of HIV/AIDS is essential for all organisations, and that external mainstreaming is a basic strategy for all humanitarian and development organisations. However, AIDS also demands specialised AIDS work, and there is a strong desire to do such work, rather than mainstreaming. Suppose that a development agency undertakes community research as part of mainstreaming HIV/AIDS in an agriculture project, and discovers three things: that AIDS-affected households are being excluded from the project; that among young people there are low levels of knowledge about the condition; and that carers for people who are bedridden with AIDS are desperately in need of support. If the agency were to adhere to the mainstreaming agenda, it would respond to the first need, and form complementary partnerships with specialist organisations which are better placed to address the remaining two needs.

However, in practice this may not be very feasible. Specialist organisations are likely to be operating already at full capacity, and there may be a great shortage of them, or even a total absence. Managers of the agriculture project have four choices.

- Prioritise their existing core work and ignore the needs for AIDS education and care, along with the many other non-agricultural needs that the project does not try to address.
- Continue with the core agriculture work, but begin to advocate for AIDS work in the area, taking the initiative in approaching specialist organisations, and perhaps offering incentives for organisations to expand their AIDS work to cover the area.

- Add limited low-cost elements of AIDS work to the core work, such as distributing leaflets about HIV transmission, and booklets about how to care for someone with AIDS at home.
- Fully begin AIDS work, opting to undertake HIV education and to support home-based care, either as separate projects, or integrated with the agricultural work.

Each of these options has advantages and disadvantages for the organisation and for different people within the community. Organisations which are mainstreaming HIV/AIDS in situations where specialist support services do not exist are likely to face some difficult decisions.

Summary

This chapter has shown a web of causes of the HIV/AIDS pandemic, derived from a view of AIDS as an issue of under-development which has four levels of determinants and related programme responses. While the web presents the whole picture, and so the whole response to AIDS, at present the global response to the problem, including that of development and humanitarian organisations, is biased towards the bio-medical and behavioural levels. This chapter has proposed that organisations are variously suited to act at different levels, and that development and humanitarian organisations should adopt mainstreaming of HIV/AIDS as their basic strategy. By doing so they can operate at the level to which they are best suited, and provide coverage in an area of the web which has been, so far, largely ignored. Table 5.2 summarises this chapter's implications for the response of development and humanitarian organisations to HIV and AIDS.

Overall, Part 1 of the book has argued that, particularly in areas with existing and increasing HIV epidemics, 'business as usual' is a limited strategy which poses many dangers. By failing to mainstream, development agencies can cause negative effects which act against development goals and the fight against HIV/AIDS. Significantly, by not mainstreaming, agencies also miss the opportunity to maximise the way in which they address HIV/AIDS indirectly, both inside and outside the organisation. At present, many development organisations with and without AIDS projects continue the bulk of their development work, and the way they run their business, as if AIDS did not exist. In a sense, by mainstreaming HIV/AIDS, all of them could continue to do what they do, but do it better. Part 2 of the book presents practical ideas for doing just that.

Table 5.2 Summary of implications for the response of development and humanitarian agencies to HIV and AIDS

Internal mainstreaming of HIV/AIDS	Necessary for all organisations in affected countries; some aspects of the process relevant to all organisations in countries with low HIV prevalence.
External mainstreaming of HIV/AIDS	The basic initial strategy for all development and humanitarian agencies in affected countries. The process could be modified – either scaled down, or focused on related issues such as gender equity – in settings with low HIV prevalence.
AIDS work (stand-alone and integrated)	An important complementary strategy for those development and humanitarian agencies with sufficient capacity to undertake both mainstreaming of HIV/AIDS and AIDS work. Those without such capacity should, where possible, form partnerships with others engaged in AIDS work.

Part 2 | Ideas for mainstreaming HIV/AIDS

6 | Strategy and guiding principles

Introduction

At present, development and humanitarian organisations have not tried out the idea of mainstreaming HIV/AIDS for long enough to have developed a body of good practice. This points to a paradox: agencies need guidelines to help them to mainstream, but they need to mainstream in order to develop guidelines. The way out of this dilemma is for individuals and agencies to apply their good sense, their wider experience, and a willingness to learn, to their experiments with mainstreaming. Their initial mistakes and tentative successes will gradually form lessons which will, in turn, inform others.

The research for *AIDS on the Agenda*, the longer book on which this one is based, brought together a range of experiences of internal and external mainstreaming of HIV/AIDS and of gender. Part 2 of this shorter book draws on those experiences to provide a set of practical ideas for mainstreaming. It is hoped that they will contribute to the on-going process of experimentation and development of the approach. More detailed suggestions about how to apply the ideas are presented in the ten user-friendly Units in the Resources section of *AIDS on the Agenda*. The Units, and the complete text of *AIDS on the Agenda*, are available and downloadable from Oxfam GB's website http://www.oxfam.org.uk/what_we_do/issues/hivaids/aidsagenda.htm.
In this text, they are referred to by number and in bold: for example, 'see Unit 2'.

This chapter presents a broad strategy which agencies might follow in order to get started, and the main options available to them. It also introduces a set of guiding principles.

Strategy

Mainstreaming, as proposed in this book, is about making development and humanitarian organisations and their work responsive and relevant to the changes brought about by HIV and AIDS. At its most simple, the essence of mainstreaming can be expressed in three questions, concerning the effects of AIDS on organisations and the people with whom they work, and the effects of the organisations' work on the people's susceptibility to HIV infection and vulnerability to the impacts of AIDS. These questions are summarised in Table 6.1.

The questions are simple, but not so the process of getting them asked, answered, and acted on systematically as part of the on-going business of development and humanitarian organisations.

Table 6.1 Mainstreaming HIV/AIDS: key questions for development and humanitarian organisations	
Internal mainstreaming	How do HIV and AIDS affect our organisation and its ability to work effectively against poverty, now and in the future?
External mainstreaming	How do HIV and AIDS affect the people we work with, in terms of their efforts to escape from poverty, now and in the future?
	How is our work making them more or less susceptible to HIV infection and more or less vulnerable to the impacts of AIDS?

Beginning the process

All change comes from somewhere. For any organisation, the initiative to mainstream HIV/AIDS could come from a variety of sources, such as personal experiences of managers or field staff; the conclusions of a programme review; a directive from head office; a funding opportunity; or the advocacy of another organisation. Whatever the source, experience suggests that if the mainstreaming process is to succeed, it needs at least one champion: someone who is interested in the idea, and who is able to learn about it, and to inspire others to become interested and involved. An initial strategy, therefore, is for a champion to establish an informal group of like-minded people who choose to join together in order to assemble the basic ingredients for a more formal process of mainstreaming HIV/AIDS. Their internal advocacy might use a variety of strategies, such as presenting the case for mainstreaming to senior management, drawing on the experience and expertise of others to influence their organisation's decision makers, or focusing efforts on influential individuals who are likely to be receptive to the idea. Whatever tactics the champions use, they will need to be persistent, and to support their arguments with facts and proposals for action.

It may be useful to note three conditions which result from successful advocacy for change: identification, ownership, and empowerment (Barnett and Whiteside 2002:321). When applied to promoting mainstreaming within an organisation, the conditions that need to be fulfilled are as follows.

- First, key members of staff need to **identify with** the issue of AIDS, and to understand its connections to poverty and under-development.

- Second, they need to **own the issue**, in the sense of believing that AIDS is relevant to the work of their organisation.

- Third, key staff need to be **empowered** to act, through recognising mainstreaming as an effective way to respond, and one which they are motivated to try.

If champions can achieve those three things among key members of staff, then the most intangible, but potent, ingredient is in place: **commitment**.

Commitment, or 'political will', among senior and influential staff seems to be a critical factor, because it will help to secure the other basic requirement for mainstreaming: **resources**. This has two elements. One is the capacity to begin and sustain mainstreaming activities. This capacity may come either from allocating or reallocating existing resources to mainstreaming – by drawing on a training budget, for example, or using in-house trainers – or from securing new resources in the form of funding for mainstreaming.

The second element is person power, because experience suggests that it is crucial to have some people with designated responsibility for mainstreaming. In larger organisations it may be possible to employ specialist staff; in all organisations, however, designated responsibility needs to be spread widely, and in this respect 'focal points' can be very useful. Staff members who are focal points do not take responsibility for mainstreaming; instead they encourage and support the process. Their role is similar to that of the champions, but with the difference that they are formally recognised and strategically placed throughout the organisation. For focal points to be effective, they need to understand and communicate their role clearly, and to be given enough time and resources to do the work, plus management support and some level of influence within the organisation. They also need the personal motivation and skills required to understand and promote the mainstreaming agenda. At the senior level, it is helpful if a key decision maker takes the lead on mainstreaming.

There are two other strategies which will encourage mainstreaming. They cannot, however, be used by individual champions: they are tools for institutions. First, agencies may encourage mainstreaming by making funds available for the process. This is a strategy used by donors, particularly with regard to mainstreaming gender-related concerns, but it could also be used to facilitate mainstreaming responses to HIV/AIDS within an organisation.

However, experience from gender mainstreaming shows that full external funding for the mainstreaming process might discourage a sense of ownership among staff. Second, donors and organisations may decide that mainstreaming is not an option but an essential activity; they may attempt to enforce such a policy through programme review, budgeting, and funding processes.

Options

Within the mainstreaming process, organisations have to decide which aspects to adopt, and what degrees of priority to give to them. The main components of the whole agenda are internal mainstreaming, mainstreaming in development work, and mainstreaming in humanitarian work. Organisations which work with partners have similar options with regard to supporting their partners. In addition, there are the options of implementing, or supporting partners to implement, direct AIDS work, and of aiming to integrate such work. And in situations of low HIV prevalence, organisations might opt for any of the elements already mentioned, or may choose to act on related issues, such as gender equality. These options are summarised in Table 6.2.

There are also choices to be made in terms of the sequence of events. An organisation with sufficient capacity might opt to undertake different components of mainstreaming simultaneously. The processes might be separate, but they might also overlap. For example, an agency could combine aspects of external mainstreaming in its own programmes with support to its partners to do likewise. The alternative is to deal with each component in turn. Although slower, this would allow experience from each component to inform the following phases. For example, an agency could incorporate the lessons learned from its own external mainstreaming into its later efforts to support its partners to do likewise. One fact emerges very clearly, however, from experience of mainstreaming gender and HIV/AIDS: awareness raising and basic training for staff is one of the first steps. It is essential to ensure a better understanding of AIDS and its personal and work implications among a critical mass of staff before proceeding to other aspects of mainstreaming.

Table 6.2 Responding to HIV/AIDS: options for development and humanitarian organisations

Internal mainstreaming of HIV and AIDS
For all organisations, including those focused on AIDS work

Supporting staff to reduce their susceptibility to HIV, and to cope better with AIDS	+	Modifying the organisation's internal procedures in the context of AIDS

External mainstreaming in development and/or humanitarian work
For all development and humanitarian organisations

Training and capacity building	+	Community research	+	Designing mainstreamed programmes	+	Adapting systems

Options for AIDS work
For all development and humanitarian organisations

Form complementary partnerships with specialist AIDS organisations	or	Fund or build capacity for other organisations to do AIDS work	or	Engage in elements of AIDS work	or	Engage fully in AIDS work

Supporting partners
For all organisations working with partners

Internal mainstreaming	+/or	External mainstreaming	+/or	AIDS work

In low-prevalence settings

Scaled-down process of internal and external mainstreaming of HIV/AIDS	or	Internal and external mainstreaming of related issues such as gender equity	+/or	The options relating to AIDS work, and to supporting partners

Guiding principles

The previous section listed some basic requirements for beginning and sustaining mainstreaming, in terms of commitment among key people, and allocation of human and financial resources. This section proposes seven principles which emerged from the case studies gathered for *AIDS on the Agenda*.

First, mainstreaming is best approached as a **learning process**. It is not a one-off event, because, even if an organisation successfully institutionalised attention to HIV/AIDS, it would still need to engage in on-going activities such as training new staff. Moreover, the context is a dynamic one, so organisations need to be alert to changes in, for example, the availability and cost of antiretroviral treatments, patterns of HIV infection within the community, and trends in the impacts of AIDS on employees and community members. Furthermore, the process involves experimentation, reflection and learning; organisations will inevitably make mistakes, and must learn from them if practice is to improve.

A second principle is that the process of mainstreaming should **involve employees as active participants**. This is very important for internal mainstreaming, because the initiatives which aim to support staff will be effective only if the staff, who are in effect 'project beneficiaries', have helped to shape their design and delivery. Consultation on controversial issues such as medical benefits, and sensitive issues such as confidentiality, is likely to be particularly important if workplace policies are to be accepted and used by employees. Staff also need to be actively engaged in activities relating to mainstreaming HIV/AIDS in programme work, because success requires changes in the hearts and minds of employees; in particular, it is crucial to develop a shared understanding and vision among employees about what mainstreaming means and what they are trying to achieve through mainstreaming. One cannot make mainstreaming happen by simply telling staff what mainstreaming is and instructing them to do it.

Related to this is the third principle: mainstreaming must **involve people who are affected by HIV and AIDS**. Mainstreaming is not an academic exercise, but one which responds to the experiences of individuals, households, and communities affected by AIDS. If organisations are to understand the implications of HIV and AIDS for their work, then as part of the process their staff need to learn directly from women, men, and children affected by the pandemic. Moreover, if organisations are to make their programme work more relevant to the changes brought about by HIV and AIDS, then they need to involve affected people in devising, implementing, and monitoring suitable adaptations to that work. Furthermore, involving people who are openly HIV-positive is a tried and tested strategy for challenging social stigma, and may, among other benefits, help organisations to promote the idea of positive living to their staff.

The fourth principle proposed here is straightforward: people who are mainstreaming HIV/AIDS need to **attend to gender-related issues** throughout the process. Gender and AIDS are always connected, such that attention to gender issues is integral to all the elements of both internal and external mainstreaming of HIV/AIDS.

The fifth principle is that organisations need to **learn from, and link with, others**. It makes sense, for example, for organisations which are undertaking internal mainstreaming to share with other agencies their training curricula, research on HIV statistics or employment law, and lessons learned, in order to reduce duplication of effort and so make the process more effective. Similarly, with regard to external mainstreaming, learning can be accelerated if agencies share with each other their experiences of what seems to work and what does not. Connected to this is the possible need for specialist help: for example, assistance with training, professional advice about employment law, help in predicting future impacts, or advice about the feasibility of particular modifications to programme work.

The sixth principle is that mainstreaming is aimed at **making changes as appropriate**, both internally and externally. In other words, unless the organisation and its work are already nearly ideal, the outcome of mainstreaming should be changes. However, these changes should be practical and plausible modifications to existing approaches, perhaps involving new initiatives within a programme, rather than a complete revolution in the way in which the agency operates. Furthermore, although the modifications are likely to aim to reduce the exclusion of AIDS-affected households from development projects, this does not mean that all activities must become completely accessible to all AIDS-affected households.

Finally, it is critical to attend to practice and to **monitor progress actively**. Policies can set out excellent ideas, but they may then be ignored or misapplied. On-going monitoring of the application of the policies, and their effects, provides the opportunity to modify and improve both policies and practice. In the same way, planned activities and changes need to be monitored, assessed, and revised as necessary, as do methods to institutionalise attention to HIV and AIDS.

Summary: principles for mainstreaming HIV/AIDS

The basic ingredients for mainstreaming are commitment, capacity (including funding), and person power. The principles are as follows:

1 Approach mainstreaming as a learning process.

2 Involve employees as active participants.

3 Involve people who are affected by HIV and AIDS.

4 Attend to gender-related issues throughout.

5 Learn from, and link with, others.

6 Make changes as appropriate.

7 Monitor actively.

The next three chapters present ideas for mainstreaming HIV/AIDS internally, then externally in development work, and externally in humanitarian programmes.

7 | Ideas for internal mainstreaming of HIV/AIDS

Internal mainstreaming is the process of changing organisational policy and practice in order to reduce both the organisation's susceptibility to HIV infection and its vulnerability to the impacts of AIDS. It has two elements: supporting staff through AIDS work, such as HIV prevention and treatment; and modifying the way in which the organisation functions: for example, in terms of workforce planning, budgeting, and ways of working.

Supporting staff to reduce their susceptibility to HIV, and to cope better with AIDS

The group of activities under this heading aim to help staff as individuals to face up to AIDS, to avoid HIV transmission, and, if infected, to manage their condition as best they can. Because the functioning of any organisation is strongly influenced by its employees' performance, effective work to support them also benefits the organisation.

Helping staff to face up to the problem

Helping staff to face up to HIV/AIDS as a personal issue means helping them to understand the condition, to consider how it relates to them, and to think through ways in which they may try to reduce their own susceptibility and vulnerability.

The most common activity among organisations responding to AIDS internally is the provision of AIDS education for employees. The impact of awareness-raising workshops can be strengthened – and measured – by first assessing the knowledge and attitudes of the participants. An easy way to do this is through an anonymous questionnaire which participants complete before the workshop, and repeat after it. The results enable trainers first to match the workshop to the participants' needs, and later to measure changes in their knowledge and attitudes. Questions might cover topics such as understanding of HIV transmission, attitudes towards people with HIV and AIDS, personal risk assessment, and willingness to talk openly about HIV (for an example, see **Unit 3** in *AIDS on the Agenda*, downloadable from http://www.oxfam.org.uk/what_we_do/issues/hivaids/aidsagenda.htm).

The effectiveness of workshops can also be increased by ensuring that staff take an active role, discussing key issues together, rather than listening passively to lectures. It is sometimes helpful for people to work in peer groups with others of the same sex or the same level of seniority. Inviting people who are openly HIV-positive to contribute to the workshop can make HIV and AIDS more real to participants, particularly in circumstances where few people are willing to talk openly about their HIV status. Hearing someone who is HIV-positive talk freely about his or her experiences and plans can also challenge stigma and provide a role model of positive living. In most cases, organisations will need to link with groups of HIV-positive people or local GIPA (Greater Involvement of People with AIDS) projects in order to find someone who is willing and able to fulfil such a role.

The most basic awareness-raising workshops typically cover facts and misunderstandings about HIV transmission; the difference between HIV and AIDS; HIV/AIDS statistics; and the methods of preventing HIV infection. For individuals and organisations to benefit more fully, however, workshops need also to cover topics such as counselling, HIV testing, and positive living. Participants might also consider their own attitudes, in particular through discussing issues of stigma and negative discrimination, as well as practical concerns such as care and support for people with AIDS.

Ideally, workshops or discussion groups should not be one-off events, but part of an on-going process, with sessions focused on themes that are important to staff members. For example, the scope could be broadened to address factors which influence susceptibility to HIV infection, such as poor inter-personal communication skills and the use of alcohol and other drugs, or topics related to vulnerability to the impacts of AIDS, including financial management and the writing of a will to make financial provision for surviving dependants. An on-going process also ensures that new staff are involved, and encourages them to reflect and learn alongside existing employees.

In addition to equipping staff with information, and giving them a chance to consider the issues, AIDS workshops may act as an occasion for consultation and problem solving. For example, imagine that at the end of a basic AIDS workshop some participants identify access to good-quality condoms as a priority, and others express interest in using counselling and testing services. In a follow-up workshop, managers could present options to staff, in order to obtain their feedback; or staff could be given the task of proposing appropriate services themselves. As experience of good development practice suggests, involving the beneficiaries in the design of a project increases its chances of success, because the project will match the needs of staff, and they will feel a greater sense of ownership of the project.

In summary, ideas for helping staff to face up to AIDS as a personal issue include the following:

- Use preliminary and follow-up questionnaires to match workshops to their needs, and to assess the impact of the sessions.

- Use active, participatory methods, rather than lecturing staff about AIDS.

- Invite people who are openly HIV-positive to take an active part in the workshops.

- Organise an on-going series of sessions, rather than one-off events.

- Arrange separate workshops or activities for employees in peer groups (same-sex groups, or people on similar levels of seniority).

- Go beyond the basics of HIV transmission to cover wider issues, according to participants' interests.

- Use workshops as an opportunity to develop other aspects of internal mainstreaming, by consulting with staff, or asking them to devise strategies.

Creating a workplace policy

For most organisations, establishing a workplace policy, or revising an existing one, is a key part of the internal mainstreaming of HIV/AIDS. This may be a policy about HIV/AIDS specifically, or a policy about chronic and terminal diseases including HIV/AIDS (which may be a fairer approach, and one which is also less likely to cause stigma). In general, workplace policies formalise the responsibilities of the organisation to its employees; they typically include employment criteria; workplace prevention activities; and benefits and treatment for infected and affected employees.

In devising or modifying a workplace policy, organisations seek to provide measures which benefit staff, and so benefit the organisation, while honouring their legal obligations. The appropriate level of benefits will depend on the organisation's staffing structure, and its employees' susceptibilities and vulnerabilities; it is therefore important to undertake research (described in the next section) into how AIDS is already affecting the organisation, and how it is likely to affect it in the future. If an organisation provides very generous benefits to employees, which are greater than the benefits that the organisation will gain, it may risk damage to its functioning and finances. Alternatively, an organisation which provides very few benefits is likely to experience high costs in the long term, including employees' absenteeism, problems in retaining staff, and, perhaps, damage to the organisation's reputation.

Devising a policy may involve research into, for example, various methods of health insurance, with the idea of offering a more flexible scheme which allows employees to determine the balance of pension and health benefits that they opt to receive. It might involve deciding to hold central funds to pay for treatment for health problems which are excluded from insurance cover, or to share costs and liabilities among programmes; it might also involve investigating the legal implications of changing employees' terms and conditions. This research may be complex and time-consuming, so organisations should ideally share their findings with other agencies in the area, to avoid duplication of effort. Organisations should also review their policies on recruitment and employment, to ensure that the organisation does not discriminate against people infected with HIV.

The process of devising or revising a workplace policy also requires consultation with employees. A first step is to learn about their experiences of HIV and AIDS, their perceptions of the main impacts that HIV/AIDS is having on the organisation, and their priorities for action (see **Unit 1** of *AIDS on the Agenda* at the website mentioned on page 61 for detailed suggestions). In areas with high HIV-prevalence rates, cost-cutting measures may be necessary, such as enforcing existing policies more strictly, reducing sick-leave allowances, or limiting the number of dependants who can be included in the organisation's health scheme. Understandably, staff are unlikely to welcome such measures. However, the changes are likely to cause less resentment if staff have been involved in the process – for example, through research into their experiences and needs – and if they understand the constraints on the organisation, and the need to protect its sustainability. It therefore makes sense to avoid raising employees' expectations, and to be open about the findings of research into predicted impact, and the reasons behind the proposed changes to the policy. On the other hand, revisions to workplace policies may work in favour of employees. For example, the organisation may decide that it is unacceptable to stipulate HIV as a condition that is excluded from its health scheme, or it may decide to provide anti-retroviral treatment to staff who need it. Employees will also benefit from having their entitlements formally recorded, rather than being subject to unpredictable decisions based on managers' discretion.

Following consultation and final revisions, organisations should issue the final policy and find ways of ensuring that staff and managers are aware of its contents; for example, by giving all staff members a leaflet summarising the main points of the policy. When implementing the policy, managers may need other resources, such as guidance on not discriminating against HIV-positive staff, or advice on practical issues such as procuring condoms.

Of course, it is important to monitor the way in which the policy is used in practice. By assessing trends over time and investigating problems –

for example, low take-up of counselling services, or medical costs that are higher than expected – it is more likely that the policy will support staff and protect the organisation's work from the impacts of AIDS. Experience shows that having a policy in place, even for several years, does not necessarily result in a supportive workplace where the impacts of HIV and AIDS are minimised. Careful follow-up is needed, to identify where problems exist and to find ways of addressing them. Some ActionAid programmes, for example, have found that hiring an openly HIV-positive member of staff (through GIPA) has helped to challenge discrimination within the workplace, and encouraged employees to go for counselling and an HIV test.

To summarise, the following suggestions could help organisations to develop workplace policies:

- Base policies on research into the current and likely impacts of AIDS on the organisation.

- Make benefits available to employees which will also benefit the organisation.

- Attend to legal obligations to employees (which may vary from country to country).

- Involve and consult with staff, and explain to them the rationale behind policy decisions.

- Make sure that managers and employees know about the policy and its contents, and support managers to implement it.

- Monitor the policy's implementation, assess its effects, and modify the policy as necessary.

Modifying the ways in which organisations function in the context of HIV/AIDS

Internal mainstreaming involves more than supporting staff members to change their behaviour, because the susceptibility and vulnerability of organisations to HIV and AIDS are also determined by the ways in which the organisations function. This section, therefore, concerns efforts by organisations to devise possible modifications to their existing systems and policies.

Learning about the current impact of AIDS on the organisation

Getting a sense of how AIDS is already affecting an organisation is a relatively simple activity which can set in motion the process of internal main-streaming. For example, the findings may help to secure the necessary commitment and resources – staff time or funding – to move on to the more complex business of predicting the impacts of HIV and AIDS, and analysing the various options for the organisation. The process also has the advantage that, as with good community work, it directly involves the staff – who will be the subjects and beneficiaries of any changes in policy and practice.

Topics for this research might include employees' sense of the organisational culture with regard to HIV and AIDS; their perceptions of the impacts that HIV and AIDS are having on the organisation; personal impacts that staff have experienced, and the consequences of those impacts for their work; perceptions of the main problems that they face in the workplace with regard to HIV/AIDS; ideas about what the organisation might do; and what their own priorities are. In terms of methodology, a mixture of face-to-face methods (such as interviews or focus-group discussions) and questionnaires is likely to be ideal.

Some organisations may also be able to supplement data gained from staff by analysing existing data on sickness leave, medical costs, and staff turn-over. Overall, the results should provide a picture of how AIDS is already affecting staff, and hence the organisation itself. The results should ideally be reported back to staff, along with information about the next steps that are proposed in the mainstreaming process.

In summary, ideas for assessing the current impacts of AIDS on the organisation include the following:

- Use an anonymous questionnaire, to obtain comparable quantitative data from a large number of staff members.

- Use face-to-face methods to get more detailed information from small numbers of staff, or from key members of staff.

- Ask staff about the impacts of AIDS on the organisation in general, and on themselves and their work in particular, and the problems that they face with regard to AIDS and the workplace.

- Extend the scope to ask for employees' ideas and priorities for action.

- Analyse existing personnel data.

- Report the findings back to employees, and tell them the next steps that the organisation is planning.

Predicting the impacts of AIDS on the organisation, and analysing the options for responding

In choosing a method for predicting the impacts of AIDS, organisations need to balance the accuracy that they want against the investment that they are able to make. A full institutional audit is a complex and time-consuming process which requires external expertise (see Barnett and Whiteside 2002:253 for an outline). It is most often used by large businesses, which can use computer modelling and HIV testing to undertake sophisticated predictions and analyses of the likely impacts of AIDS on their profits, and the cost-effectiveness of various ways of responding.

For other organisations, such as NGOs, which do not measure their success in terms of profit and loss, a more basic and less costly method is likely to be more appropriate. However, there is little guidance available to them that is specific to their needs. The process described here is a basic approach to predicting the impact of HIV and AIDS, which can be undertaken without the expense of hiring external experts. A simple example is given, to illustrate the process, in Tables 7.1 to 7.3. It is presented with caution, however, because although it is based on the experiences of Oxfam GB, it has not been tried and tested over several years. And, as with all models, it may be of little use to small organisations, where the small number of employees makes predicted impacts highly questionable.

The starting point is to assess the rate of HIV prevalence and cases of AIDS within the organisation over a period of time, perhaps five or ten years. This is done by taking the number of employees and applying assumptions about the rate of HIV among them; the proportion of HIV-positive staff who are in the final stage of HIV infection (suffering from AIDS); and how many of the employees with AIDS leave the organisation each year. Table 7.1 shows an example of a fictional organisation with 100 employees, which finds that three of its staff may develop AIDS each year.

The next stage is to consider the direct financial costs to the organisation, such as health-care costs. One must build in assumptions about the average costs incurred for employees who do not have AIDS, and those incurred by staff with AIDS. Table 7.2 shows this stage for the organisation featured in Table 7.1. The calculations suggest that its health costs will be seven per cent higher than they would have been without AIDS.

Table 7.1 Predicting the prevalence of HIV and AIDS within an organisation

Predicting HIV and AIDS prevalence within the organisation	Employees	Notes
A: number of employees	100	
B: assumed proportion of employees who are HIV+	20%	National prevalence is 20%
A x B = **C:** estimated number of HIV+ employees	20	
D: assumed proportion of HIV+ employees with AIDS	15%	National average is 15%
C x D = **E: estimated number of employees developing AIDS each year**	3.0	

Table 7.2 Predicting the direct costs of health care for employees with AIDS

Predicting the direct cost of health care	Currency units	Notes
F: maximum allowable health costs per employee	1,000	
A x (30% of F) = **G:** likely health costs, without AIDS	30,000	Assume average employee uses 30% of allowable health costs
(A - E) x (30% of F) = **H:** likely health costs for employees who do not have AIDS	29,100	
E x F = **I:** likely health costs for employees with AIDS	3,000	Assume staff with AIDS will use 100% of allowable health costs
(H +I - G)/G x 100 = **estimated percentage increase in health costs as a result of AIDS**	7%	

The final stage concerns the indirect costs to the organisation, such as the impacts of AIDS on staff absences from work. By making assumptions about the amount of leave taken on average by staff who do not have AIDS, and the amount taken by staff with AIDS, one can estimate the effect that AIDS might have on overall levels of absenteeism. Table 7.3 suggests that the organisation will experience ten per cent more days of staff absence than it would have done without AIDS.

Table 7.3 Predicting the indirect cost of absenteeism

Predicting the indirect cost of absenteeism	Days	Notes
J: maximum allowable days' paid sick leave per employee per year	50	Average employee uses 50% of this
K: maximum allowable days' unpaid leave per employee per year	60	Average employee uses none of this
A x (50% of J) = **L:** likely absenteeism, without AIDS	2,500	
(A - E) x (50% of J) = **M:** likely absenteeism among employees who do not have AIDS	2,425	
(E x J) + (E x K) = **N:** likely absenteeism among employees with AIDS	330	Assume staff with AIDS will take 100% of allowable sick leave and unpaid leave
(M + N - L)/L x 100 = **estimated percentage increase in absenteeism as a result of AIDS**	10%	

The example illustrated in Tables 7.1 to 7.3 is a very simple one. It deals only with employees, one form of benefit, and two forms of absenteeism, and it covers only one year. The calculations could be made more complex, to reflect more closely the situation in a real organisation, in the following ways:

- Add extra columns to predict impact over more than one year. The calculations would need to make allowance for any likely changes over time, such as the effects of inflation, or predicted changes in HIV prevalence. (In **Unit 2** of *AIDS on the Agenda*, downloadable from the website mentioned on page 61, the same calculations are shown for a five-year period.)

- For a large organisation, it may be appropriate to introduce different assumptions about levels of HIV prevalence for different types of staff.

- Take account of costs incurred where employees are HIV-positive and becoming sick periodically, but not yet suffering from AIDS.

- Include employees' dependants in the figures, if they are covered by the organisation's benefit schemes.

- Include other direct costs, such as terminal benefits which are paid when an employee dies or retires due to ill-health.

- Include other indirect costs, such as those for recruiting and training staff to replace those who leave due to AIDS, or absenteeism due to staff members taking time off to care for dependants with AIDS.

Because the calculations are based on many assumptions, those assumptions have a big effect on the predictions. Once the calculations are set up as a spreadsheet, different assumptions can be put in, to generate different scenarios, such as worst-case and best-case predictions. The spreadsheet can also be used to explore the effects of changing variables: for example, the number of dependants per employee who are entitled to receive benefits from the organisation. Parallel spreadsheets can also be used to explore the costs and benefits of options such as providing antiretroviral treatment for employees and/or their dependants.

The process of doing such calculations might be the responsibility of one or a few members of staff, but it is important that a wider range of staff should be consulted. Information may need to be obtained from outside the organisation: for example, data about local HIV-prevalence rates, and the length of time that an employee with AIDS may continue to serve the organisation, according to the various treatment options.

The quantitative findings of such an impact assessment might also be combined with research into current impacts of AIDS on staff, to consider future impacts on unquantified factors such as quality of work, loss of experience, and staff morale. The findings of both forms of research – the impacts already experienced, and the impacts that are predicted – can then inform, and be used to support the case for, other aspects of internal mainstreaming of HIV/AIDS, in particular the formulation or revision of a workplace policy.

In summary, ideas for predicting the internal impacts of AIDS include the following:

- Select a method which suits your organisation's needs, in terms of the cost of the exercise and the accuracy of the outcome.

- Allocate responsibility to one or a few members of staff, but involve others in the process.

- Adapt models to fit the organisation and its most relevant variables, seeking external assistance where necessary to make informed assumptions.

- Use the calculations to explore a range of options which the organisation could adopt.

- Use the findings for internal consultation and consideration, and creating or modifying a workplace policy.

Changing policy and practice

The main outcome of the research described above should be a new or revised workplace policy which, if implemented effectively, will help to reduce the organisation's susceptibility to HIV infection and vulnerability to the impacts of AIDS. As a result, for example, HIV-positive staff might be enabled to work and contribute to the organisation for longer; or absenteeism might be reduced by introducing rules about taking leave for funerals. Beyond the changes in workplace policies, however, organisations also need to examine the ways in which they function, with a particular emphasis on ways in which that functioning may be unintentionally making the organisation more susceptible and vulnerable. This is similar to the way in which external mainstreaming requires an organisation to assess its programme work, and to try to minimise the negative consequences which it may be having on community members' susceptibility and vulnerability.

Staff members may be more susceptible to HIV infection by virtue of their employment by the organisation. For example, health-sector staff face the occupational hazard of HIV infection through a needle-stick injury. This kind of susceptibility can be reduced by the provision of correct equipment, and adherence to safe procedures such as careful handling and disposal of injection equipment. In the event of a needle-stick injury, or a rape, organisations should quickly provide access to antiretroviral drugs, which can sometimes stop a person becoming HIV-positive after he or she has been exposed to HIV.

Some of the employment-related factors which may increase susceptibility to HIV may, however, be difficult to change. For example, some staff may need to travel regularly, and may have casual sexual relations when they are away from their families. It may be possible to reduce the number of trips by means of better planning, use of information technology, or decentralisation of responsibilities. However, in organisations whose offices are widely spread, the need to travel cannot be eliminated. An organisation can supply its staff with good-quality condoms for men and women, but it is the responsibility of individuals to use them consistently, or to refrain from sexual relations altogether.

Staff may also be more susceptible to HIV infection if they are posted away from home. Chapter 4 cited an example from Ghana, where teachers were unintentionally made more susceptible because their salaries were often not paid on time. For female staff who are posted away from their support networks, the simple measure of ensuring that they are paid regularly should reduce their need to seek financial support and engage in sexual bargaining. Another possibility is to allow staff regular 'long weekends' at home. This particularly applies to people working in intensive emergency situations, where measures such as respite breaks, counselling, and debriefing can help them to maintain mental health, and so be less likely to use unsafe sex as a coping mechanism. Such a measure might not involve extra expense, if employees were allowed to 'save up' hours of overtime work and then take off days in lieu. In stable settings, a more radical response would be to enable employees to have their families living with them at their posting: for example, suitable accommodation might be provided for teachers and their families. To conclude, it is important to assess, with staff members, whether ways of working are making them more susceptible to HIV infection, and to take reasonable measures to minimise the risks.

With regard to reducing the organisation's vulnerability to the impacts of AIDS, this chapter has already considered efforts focused on support for employees. The idea of modifying the organisation's mode of functioning is concerned with changing policy and practice. After all, however good the organisation's HIV-prevention work, in highly affected countries all but the smallest organisations can be sure of having HIV-positive staff. But there are few experiences of this on which to draw. Instead, this section reviews some possible options, all related to human-resource and finance functions.

Human resources

For human-resource departments, the main step is to consider future staffing needs in the light of the predicted impacts of AIDS on employees. If problems are expected, such as shortages of skilled staff (especially frontline professionals such as teachers, health workers, or agriculturalists), or higher levels of staff turn-over, the agency should take the initiative to reduce their impacts; for example,

- by taking measures to retain existing staff, or to attract back professionals who have left or retired;
- offering on-the-job training if it is not possible to recruit qualified people;
- promoting career development within the organisation;
- and shifting from long and expensive training courses for a minority of staff to on-going capacity building for all staff, using short courses with rapid results.

It may also be possible to improve the functioning of the human-resources department, by investing in it in order to, for example, speed up recruitment procedures and strengthen the provision of training.

To reduce the impact of absenteeism, the organisation could also consider

- organising its staff to work in teams;
- arranging for people to share responsibilities;
- and documenting each post-holder's main work practices.

Such measures are particularly important in the case of key posts, where the absence of the post-holder would have a disproportionate and serious impact on the organisation. In cases where disruption can be predicted, for example if a staff member falls ill repeatedly, or declares his or her HIV-positive status, additional efforts may further ease the impact. These might include

- arranging temporary cover (including paid overtime by existing staff);
- encouraging hand-over of information and transfer of skills;
- and reducing stress on the staff member by reducing his or her workload.

All of these tasks become more feasible if the organisation encourages a culture in which HIV-positive employees are willing to declare their HIV status.

Finance

In terms of finance, the task is to include HIV/AIDS in budgets, and to get those budgets funded. Having predicted future impacts, and agreed the workplace policy, it is necessary to fit all the expected costs into the organisation's budgeting. This will involve adjusting budgets related to staff salaries and benefits, and initiatives such as awareness-raising workshops, provision of condoms, counselling and testing, and health care. The budgets should also include the expected costs of reducing susceptibility and vulnerability to HIV and AIDS, inasmuch as an organisation intends to make any of the changes outlined above. For example, there would certainly be budgetary implications if an agency were to begin to provide staff with accommodation for themselves and their families. If an organisation is also embarking on mainstreaming HIV/AIDS in external programmes, there will, of course, be additional budgetary provisions to make.

Monitoring costs and trends

For both human resources and finances, organisations need to develop monitoring systems which will allow them to track and analyse costs and trends associated with AIDS and with internal mainstreaming over time. For example, medical costs could be tracked by monitoring

- average medical costs per employee;
- the percentage of employees incurring the maximum allowable medical costs;
- costs exceeding a certain level;
- or total medical costs expressed as a percentage of the cost of all salaries.

If it is possible without disclosing confidential information to gather data on the medical costs incurred by employees who have declared themselves to be HIV-positive, then that information would be useful in enabling more accurate planning and predictions of the financial impacts of AIDS on the organisation. Each organisation needs to develop indicators which are appropriate for its situation (see **Unit 5** of *AIDS on the Agenda* at the website mentioned on page 61 for some suggested key indicators). This may involve adjusting the organisation of budgets and accounts, so that trends in key indicators become evident. Monitoring is likely to be particularly important for managers in large or decentralised organisations, where the impacts of AIDS and responses to it may not otherwise be apparent. In addition to helping with strategic planning, and with refining internal mainstreaming processes, organisations can use their monitoring data for external advocacy; for example, to encourage other organisations to mainstream HIV/AIDS internally, and to help donors to understand the need for additional funding.

In summary, ideas for changing policy and practice include the following:

- Investigate ways in which employees' susceptibility to HIV infection may be heightened because of their jobs and because of the ways in which the organisation functions.

- Act within reason to reduce that susceptibility, by modifying policy and practice.

- Look for ways in which the organisation's functioning makes it more vulnerable to the impacts of AIDS.

- Act to reduce that vulnerability, particularly within the spheres of human-resource policy and practice, and financial-management systems.

- Identify key indicators, and actively monitor trends for both the impacts of AIDS and the impact of initiatives undertaken as part of internal mainstreaming of HIV/AIDS.

Summary

This chapter has presented ideas for the internal mainstreaming of HIV/AIDS under two headings: supporting staff, and modifying the ways in which the organisation functions. Figure 7.1 brings together all these ideas in the form of a flow chart.

Figure 7.1 Summary of key steps in internal mainstreaming

Learning about the current impacts of AIDS on the organisation

Methodology
- Anonymous questionnaire to staff
- +/or face-to-face discussions with staff or groups of staff
- +/or interviews with key staff

Scope
- Focus only on staff experiences of AIDS and impacts on their work.
- Or extend questioning to include their ideas and priorities for action.

Undertake research, including analysis of any existing relevant personnel data.

Report on current impacts (and staff ideas and priorities).

Feedback to employees, with next steps in the process outlined.

Use in internal advocacy for next steps in internal mainstreaming.

Predicting the impacts of AIDS on the organisation

Methodology
- Full institutional audit, with expert help, and possibility of voluntary HIV-testing of employees.
- Or in-house process, using existing computer models, or devising one for the organisation.

Scope
- Number of years to cover.
- Which variables to include (e.g. health costs, other benefits, leave taken).
- In the case of large organisations, which offices or regions to include.

Gather data, make assumptions, and do calculations.

Create a range of scenarios, e.g. 'best case' and 'worse case'.

Explore the costs and benefits of altering variables and of treatment options.

Report on predicted impacts and recommendations for action.

Internal consultation and consideration

Figure 7.1 *continued*

Devising or adapting a workplace policy

Research options e.g. flexible health insurance, or cost-sharing within an organisation.	Ensure that the policy meets legal obligations to employees.	Engage in process of consultation and modification as appropriate.

Policy which covers employment criteria; workplace prevention activities; benefits and treatment for HIV-positive and HIV-affected employees

Disseminate policy and support managers to implement it.

Monitor implementation, and modify as appropriate.

+

Modifying how the organisation functions in the context of AIDS

Susceptibility to HIV infection Identify ways in which susceptibility of employees may be heightened by virtue of working for the organisation.	*Vulnerability to the impacts of AIDS* Identify ways in which policy and practice increase the organisation's vulnerability.

Within reason, alter systems and ways of working to reduce unintended effects on employees' susceptibility.	Alter systems and ways of working in order to help the organisation to cope better with the impacts of AIDS.

Monitor implementation, and modify as appropriate.

8 | Ideas for mainstreaming HIV/AIDS in development work

The aim of mainstreaming HIV/AIDS in development work is to adapt the work in order to take into account susceptibility to HIV transmission and vulnerability to the impacts of AIDS. The focus is on core programme work in the changing context created by AIDS, ensuring that new and existing projects are relevant to that context and that they contribute positively to the wider response to HIV and AIDS. This chapter considers ideas relating to four main steps for external mainstreaming in development work:

- training and capacity building
- community research
- designing development work which indirectly addresses HIV and AIDS
- adapting systems.

Training and capacity building

Training is the first activity in the process of external mainstreaming. It is needed because staff who are not AIDS workers – such as agriculturalists, educationalists, or community-development workers – are very unlikely to feel able (or be able) to respond to the problem through their normal work. If asked to consider doing so, they are almost certain to think of doing AIDS education or other forms of AIDS work, or to resist the idea that they should address the problem at all. Both of these reactions hinder the process of mainstreaming.

Table 8.1 suggests the main components of a training course in external mainstreaming (for more detail, and some ideas for measuring the impact of such a training, see **Unit 6** of *AIDS on the Agenda*, available from http://www.oxfam.org.uk/what_we_do/issues/hivaids/aidsagenda.htm).

Table 8.1 Themes and activities for training for external mainstreaming of HIV/AIDS

Theme	Activity
Understanding the links between development and AIDS	Analysing case studies to reveal: • the complex causes of susceptibility to HIV infection (see Chapter 2); • the reinforcing cycle of causes and consequences (see Figure 2.1); • the link between gender and HIV/AIDS (see Chapter 2).
Understanding the meaning of external mainstreaming of HIV/AIDS	Using examples to explore the difference between AIDS work and mainstreaming HIV/AIDS (see Chapter 3). Thinking about the web of influences on HIV, and how different organisations are suited to act on different levels within the web (see Figure 5.1 and Table 5.1).
Learning how to undertake external mainstreaming of HIV/AIDS	Understanding the core questions for external mainstreaming of HIV/AIDS (see next sections). Talking about the next steps: undertaking community research, and modifying development programmes.

Note that participants need to have attended basic AIDS-awareness workshops before they take part in sessions about external mainstreaming.

Community research

Although the links between AIDS and development can be explained through training, this is no substitute for employees learning for themselves, at first hand, from people who are affected by AIDS, and learning about the various levels of vulnerability involved. Furthermore, community research is essential to learning about susceptibility and vulnerability in context, rather than assuming that general narratives – such as those contained in this book – apply in particular circumstances. For example, this book states that members of vulnerable, AIDS-affected households are generally less able to participate in development projects, but agencies need to discover whether or not that is true in each particular context.

The community-research element of external mainstreaming involves meeting with people of varying ages from the project area, including men, women, and older children, who have been affected by HIV and AIDS. This section does not give comprehensive guidelines on undertaking research with community members, but it provides some ideas concerning methods and contents of research in connection with mainstreaming (more detail is available in **Unit 7** of *AIDS on the Agenda*). The text assumes that the mainstreaming agenda is being applied to an existing project, but the ideas could be adapted for use in preliminary planning for a new project, allowing HIV/AIDS to be mainstreamed within it from the outset.

How to do the research, and with whom

In terms of methodology, qualitative methods are most appropriate. They could be simple discussions, guided by a series of open questions; or participatory exercises which encourage participants jointly to analyse their problems and experiences.

The most important differences within a community are likely to be sex, age, and socio-economic situation. To obtain general information, the researchers could work with peer groups, where the participants are of the same sex and at the same life stage as each other (a group of young men, for example). Listening to peer groups is often more revealing than asking questions of a mixed group: in full community meetings, age and status mean that some voices tend to predominate (older men, for example) at the expense of others (such as younger women). On specific and sensitive topics, such as the experience of having someone with AIDS in the family, the discussions should involve small numbers of affected people. Researchers need to meet with women and men, and to be alert to situations where individuals might prefer to talk privately. For these discussions, researchers could aim to meet with people who are affected in differing ways – such as care givers, grandparents looking after orphaned grandchildren, and widows – and should deliberately seek out those who are less able to participate in community meetings and group-based activities.

Topics for research

The research might begin by assessing perceptions of levels of illness and death, and the relative significance of various health problems. The focus could then move on to HIV/AIDS in particular or, if the topic seems too sensitive, to chronic illnesses in general. For peer groups, topics might include the following:

- attitudes towards men and women who are thought to have AIDS;
- the number of households thought to have been affected;
- the effects on particular types of household, their individual members, and their livelihoods;
- trends in the impacts of AIDS on households and the community level; and
- changes in attitudes towards AIDS and people with AIDS.

Discussions with HIV-positive individuals or small groups of affected women and men should focus on their experiences of chronic illness, such as the various stages that they have been through, the impacts of illness on various members of the household, and the ways in which they have responded. Researchers must be careful not to refer to AIDS by name unless the respondents themselves use the term; they should respect the fact that respondents may be willing to talk only in general terms.

An alternative theme for research would be susceptibility to HIV, considering such aspects as beliefs about the causes of AIDS and means of protection from it, and general perceptions of sexual behaviour.

From these general themes, the research can then move on to the connections between HIV/AIDS and the organisation's development work. The aim is not a full evaluation of the development work by community members, but to answer the question: *is the project reducing or increasing susceptibility and vulnerability* – a subject which can be approached in four ways, as presented in Table 8.2.

With these indications in mind, the starting point for community research is to explore each peer group's experience of the project, and its impacts on various people's lives. This could be done through guided discussion, which may be more fruitful if combined with a visual method such as a 'spider diagram' to encourage the groups to debate and analyse their views and experiences. How to do this will depend on the project's aims and activities, and the length of time since it was established. The researchers would need to devise their method, or methods, in advance (some suggestions are given in **Unit 7** of *AIDS on the Agenda*). Possible topics include the following:

- Who is participating, how, and with what consequences?
- Who is not participating, why, and with what consequences?
- Who holds power and decision-making authority within the project, and with what consequences?

Throughout the process, it is important for researchers to be alert to gender-related issues, and to AIDS-related questions, and to prompt interviewees accordingly if, for example, the consequences for women or destitute families or AIDS-affected households are not mentioned spontaneously. Researchers also need to be aware that women and girls may be subject to demands for sexual favours in return for access to project benefits.

The scope of the community research could also be extended to include asking peer groups and affected individuals to suggest ways in which the project could be improved. For example, if the research has revealed ways in which the project is hindering the fight against HIV/AIDS, by increasing susceptibility or vulnerability, then it would be valuable to generate ideas on how to minimise those unintended negative effects. However, researchers

Table 8.2 Signs of whether a project is reducing or increasing susceptibility and vulnerability

✓ Signs that the project is helping to address HIV/ AIDS indirectly	x Signs that the project is unintentionally hindering efforts to address HIV/ AIDS
Indications of helping to reduce susceptibility to HIV infection:	**Indications of hindering by increasing susceptibility to HIV infection:**
• empowerment of the poor; • improvements in women's status; • reductions in poverty levels; • greater gender equality; • reductions in migration; • and improvements in health, particularly sexual health.	• greater gender inequality; • shifts in power (e.g. decision-making and control of resources) towards men; • exclusion of poor or marginalised people, particularly women; • increased spending on alcohol, other recreational drugs, or sex; • increased mobility or migration; • unsafe sex between community members and development workers; • and sexual trading or sexual abuse of women in return for project benefits.
Indications of helping to reduce vulnerability to the impacts of AIDS:	**Indications of hindering by increasing vulnerability to the impacts of AIDS:**
• poor and vulnerable households – including those headed by women, older people, and orphans, and those with a high proportion of dependants – are participating and benefiting; • the project is reducing poverty and helping households, and particularly poor ones, to build up their assets; • the project is building the capacity of community institutions to respond to development problems, so that the community is less vulnerable to the impacts of AIDS, and more able to help those who are badly affected.	• exclusion (and stigmatisation) of poor and vulnerable households – including those headed by women, older people, and orphans, and those with a high proportion of dependants – at any stage of the project cycle; • activities in which such households 'fail' because the activities are unsuited to them; • and methods based on inputs of labour and capital which are unsustainable in the case of external shocks such as chronic illness.

should take care not to raise people's expectations: the discussions would need, at this stage, to be concerned with ideas rather than definite plans for action.

Overall, if the research shows that AIDS is having significant impacts, and that there are links between HIV/AIDS and the development project, then the research should assist the external mainstreaming process in four ways. First, the staff who act as researchers should gain a better understanding of how the pandemic is affecting the communities whom they serve, and how it is relevant to their work. Second, the staff should be more motivated to address the problem indirectly through modifying their ways of working. Third, they will be better placed to negotiate and discuss possible project modifications with community members. Fourth, the findings of community research can be used to support advocacy for mainstreaming HIV/AIDS and for AIDS work, particularly if they are well documented.

In summary, ideas for community research, conducted as part of the external mainstreaming of HIV/AIDS, include the following:

- Use discussions and participatory methods with peer groups of people, and with individuals or small numbers of people affected by AIDS or chronic illness.

- First focus on themes related to susceptibility to HIV infection, and to the impacts of AIDS, paying attention to gender, and to the implications for vulnerable people, throughout the process.

- Then move on to discuss the development project, or the planned project, with a view to identifying ways in which it may help or hinder community members' susceptibility to HIV and vulnerability to the impacts of AIDS.

- Consider extending the research to identify ways in which the project might be designed or modified to maximise its indirect positive impact on HIV and AIDS.

Designing development work which indirectly addresses HIV and AIDS

This section brings us to the purpose of external mainstreaming, which is to modify existing development work, or design new development work, so as to improve the way in which it indirectly addresses HIV and AIDS. This part of the process is based on the findings of the community research. It aims to make practical changes to existing development approaches. Staff may have valid ideas and enthusiasm for AIDS work, on which the agency may be able to act. However, these ideas should not divert all attention away from discussion of how to ensure that the organisation's core business can be made more relevant to the challenges of HIV and AIDS, and so play a greater role in the overall response to them. For the external mainstreaming process to keep moving in the right direction, the task must be to continue with, but improve, core work.

The precise process for designing 'mainstreamed' work, or modifying existing work, will depend on circumstances. For example, for a small project it may be possible to bring together all staff and stakeholders, including community representatives, to discuss the research findings, and to agree on some strategies or modifications. For a larger and more complex project, it might be appropriate for a working group of staff, stakeholders, and community representatives to develop some proposals, which would then be sent out for wider consultation and revision at community level before they were tried.

In all circumstances, however, the starting point is the findings of the community research, which should be able to answer the two questions at the heart of the external mainstreaming process:

- How do HIV and AIDS affect the people with whom we work, in terms of their efforts to escape from poverty, now and in the future?

- How is our work helping or hindering them to avoid HIV infection and to cope with the impacts of AIDS?

Although the modifications should be unique to each project, it may be helpful here to review some general ideas.

How households cope with shocks, and their implications for development work

Studies of households and their livelihoods explain household coping behaviour in two stages. (Note that the term 'coping' is not very accurate; as the following description makes clear, some households do not cope, and they disintegrate.)

First, 'pre-emptive' measures to reduce their vulnerability; in other words, things which people do in advance of a shock such as illness or crop failure to reduce the impact that it might have on their livelihoods and quality of life; for example, building up their protective assets, including savings and things such as livestock, jewellery, and household goods which can be sold if the need arises. Or, on the social side, preserving and investing in relationships with relatives and community members, who will help the household if the members need support. Another pre-emptive measure is to engage in a wider range of agricultural and other income-earning activities – so that if one fails, the household will still have some income from the others. Another measure is to choose low-risk income-generating activities which earn modest, but steady, returns.

Second, in the event of a shock of some kind, households use 'reactive' measures to manage the impact. These reactive measures fall into three phases (as already illustrated in Table 2.1). In Phase 1 the strategies are reversible: a household uses its protective assets, such as spending its savings, borrowing money from friends, or reducing expenditure on non-essential goods and services. In time, the household should be able to recover from the shock, gradually building up its savings once more and repaying its debts. However, if a household uses up all its protective assets, and cannot reduce its expenditure any further, it is forced to move to Phase 2. Now it may resort to selling productive assets (things which it uses in its agricultural and other income-earning activities, such as land or tools), or to borrowing money at very high interest rates. These strategies are difficult to reverse, because they reduce the household's capacity to generate income and to grow food, while its debts grow rapidly. If a household uses up all its productive assets, it enters Phase 3, a state of destitution, where households disintegrate, rely on charity, or migrate.

Clearly, when having to cope with a shock such as AIDS, households want to avoid Phases 2 and 3 by staying within Phase 1. And a household's ability to stay within Phase 1 depends on the success or otherwise of its pre-emptive efforts to reduce its vulnerability.

These insights provide important lessons for interventions by development agencies, which are summarised in Table 8.3. They suggest that development work with AIDS-affected communities, or communities which are not yet badly affected, should focus on supporting households' pre-emptive strategies; for example, initiatives to help to improve and maintain income flows, and to plan for future shocks by building up assets. These can be characterised as methods to **strengthen households' safety-nets**, which reduce vulnerability to the impacts of AIDS; they are likely to have the additional benefit of reducing susceptibility to HIV infection. In communities which are already affected, work should also aim to support affected households to remain within Phase 1, the reactive coping strategies.

However, by the time a household has reached the third phase – destitution – it has fallen through its own safety-net and is relying on whatever support is available from the community. In such circumstances, where the household has little scope for participation in general development work, it seems to be more appropriate for agencies to think in terms of **supporting community safety-nets**, in order to provide relief to destitute households; for example, AIDS projects supporting community efforts to give practical assistance to badly affected households. This kind of assistance may also help to prevent households in Phase 2 from slipping into the destitution of Phase 3.

Clearly, the strategy of strengthening household safety-nets falls within the remit of general development work, while that of strengthening community safety-nets is harder to categorise. It does involve community development work, in terms of supporting the capacity of the community to respond, but the mode is one of relief or welfare-based AIDS work. As such, it provides an example of how the overall response to HIV and AIDS requires both levels of

Table 8.3 Summary of household coping strategies and their implications for development work

Household coping mechanisms	Development-agency interventions
Pre-emptive strategies to reduce vulnerability.	Strengthen households' safety-nets, e.g. • improving incomes and income flows • encouraging saving and accumulation of assets
Reactive coping strategies: Phase 1 (reversible, using protective assets)	• avoiding use of productive assets
Phase 2 (difficult to reverse, using productive assets)	Strengthen community safety-nets, e.g. providing • help in caring for children
Phase 3 (destitution)	• food, or help in growing food • goods such as clothes and soap

(Source: adapted from Donahue 2002, and reproduced with the permission of the author)

work: development work with HIV/AIDS mainstreamed in it, and AIDS work. The following sections, discussing the mainstreaming of HIV/AIDS in development work, mainly correspond with efforts to strengthen household safety-nets, working with households that are 'vulnerable but viable'.

Agriculture

NGOs considering mainstreaming HIV/AIDS within agriculture programmes usually assume that they should do more work with households whose food supplies are insecure, which may include those headed by elderly people, women, and children. From this stems the idea that programmes should promote modified or new methods which are more suited to those households' needs and options. These methods are likely to be labour-saving, low-input, and low-risk strategies; they may arise from people's own risk-reduction strategies, and include the following:

- the use of threshing machines, mills, wheelbarrows, and carts, to reduce demands on labour-constrained households;
- tools and techniques which are better suited to elderly, weak, or young people, such as using a donkey with a special plough rather than oxen for ploughing;
- livestock which is better suited to vulnerable households: for example, for milk production, goats are cheaper and easier to handle than cows, while rabbits, chickens, and guinea fowl are easier than larger livestock to look after, but can reproduce more rapidly, and are a more divisible asset;

- inter-cropping to reduce time spent on weeding;
- mulching and minimum-tillage methods to reduce time spent on ploughing;
- more production located right outside the home, such as kitchen gardens, fruit trees, rabbits and poultry in hutches, and zero grazing for dairy cows;
- composting, mulching, and application of manure or ashes from burning crop residues to increase production without the expense of chemicals;
- inter-cropping with nitrogen-fixing plants, bunding, and 'live fences' to limit erosion and help to maintain soil fertility;
- reasonably nutritious: for example, 'survival crops' which AIDS-affected households are already using, or tree crops yielding fruit and nuts within one or two years of planting.

Note that the above suggestions are in addition to general ideas for programmes to improve food security, such as planting trees which yield fruit over a long period of the year, measures to improve the storage of food, and promoting processing and marketing initiatives to increase the earning potential of crops.

The potential modifications and their suitability will depend on the current activities of any programme, and on local farming systems. Note, however, that the common focus of the ideas suggested above is on sustainable livelihoods and improved nutrition for vulnerable people through modest but achievable forms of production, in accordance with their own risk-reduction strategies. This is contrary to the predominant focus in agricultural policy on trying to increase production rates and profit through 'high-tech' and high-status methods. So organisations wishing to promote sustainable livelihoods must not only experiment with ideas such as those presented here, but also prove their effectiveness in order to argue for policy change.

Micro-finance

Micro-finance projects, or savings and credit schemes, can help households to increase their incomes and to build up their assets, so reducing their vulnerability and, particularly for women, lowering their susceptibility to HIV infection by reducing the need to exchange sex for favours. Such projects are particularly appropriate for directing support to vulnerable households, because the loans are very small and so encourage the participation of the poor, whose short-term trading activities easily benefit from injections of small amounts of money. The gains made are likely to be modest, but may be sufficient to make a difference in quality of life, and to improve resilience to survive crises.

The following suggestions aim to make micro-finance schemes more responsive to members' needs in the context of HIV/AIDS:

- Changing the rules so that members who are sick or caring for someone else are not expelled; allowing them to miss meetings, so long as payments are made, to take a rest between loan cycles but retain their membership, or to take out a smaller loan without being penalised by a reduction in the size of future loans.

- Introducing a rule to protect the savings of married female members, which may otherwise be acquired by their husbands' relatives if they are widowed.

- Setting up a simple community bank so that people who are excluded from credit schemes because they are too economically vulnerable can save money and, in time, gain access to the credit facilities of the micro-finance service.

Micro-finance schemes do work in communities which are seriously affected by AIDS; but they should not give preferential treatment, such as lower interest rates, to members who are affected by AIDS, because the financial sustainability of the scheme could be affected if a lot of people are paying lower interest rates. Preferential treatment also tends to create resentment among other members, damaging the sense of mutual support that is needed for groups to flourish. (In any case, groups commonly devise their own ways of supporting members in times of crises, for example by making grants or loans from an emergency fund.) Nor is it recommended to form special savings and credit groups for people who are HIV-positive, because the risk of default – which is ordinarily spread among members – is too high in a group in which all the members are particularly vulnerable. In general, with regard to HIV/AIDS, micro-finance services are best positioned to serve those who are not yet badly affected (but who may well be supporting others who are affected), and to help them to reduce their vulnerability to the impacts of AIDS if it hits them. Micro-finance is not, however, an intervention that will pull destitute households out of poverty. As discussed earlier in this chapter, the phase of destitution seems to require welfare support through strengthening community safety-nets.

Allied to micro-finance is the idea of support for group-based micro-enterprises or income-generating activities. This strategy is used by NGOs and ASOs to help groups of HIV-positive people to raise money, and to help community groups to raise money to fund safety-net projects for people affected by AIDS. However, group businesses carry high risks of failure and find it difficult to generate a significant profit; even among the successes, many organisations have had disappointing experiences in this respect. Sometimes the successes are measured in terms of mutual support among members, rather than in increased income; the cost-effectiveness of such projects is rarely considered. In general, it appears that loans targeted at individuals, and in particular at women, are more effective in terms of raising incomes, improving quality of life, strengthening household safety-nets, and so reducing susceptibility and vulnerability.

Primary health care

In general, the primary health-care sector already works indirectly to reduce susceptibility to HIV and vulnerability to the impacts of AIDS by improving the health status of community members. It does this by, for example, helping to maintain people's immune systems, treating STIs, and enabling people who are ill to recover and return to work, so protecting their livelihoods. However, there may be ways in which health-care services have a more direct impact on susceptibility and vulnerability. For example, family-planning services should emphasise the option of condoms, and their benefits in terms of protecting against HIV infection, among the choices presented to prevent conception. And primary health-care providers must not deter people from seeking treatment by displaying negative attitudes towards poor people in general or, more specifically, young people or unmarried women with STIs or unplanned pregnancies. Health services may also exclude poor people through charging unaffordable fees for treatment, a problem which might be dealt with informally by exempting particularly vulnerable patients from payment, or by establishing formal safety-nets.

In terms of vulnerability to the impacts of AIDS, HIV-positive people and their families are made more vulnerable when health staff conceal the diagnosis from them, or do not explain what it means. Good and well-given advice about positive living can help people with AIDS to prioritise appropriate treatment, rest, and foods, rather than exhausting their resources in the false expectation of a full recovery. Moreover, it could be argued that the practice of omitting AIDS as one of the causes of death on death certificates contributes to the prevailing culture of denial about AIDS, and so increases susceptibility and vulnerability in the community.

Water and sanitation

In terms of HIV transmission, the main risk in water and sanitation projects seems to be the potential for sexual bargaining over access to the facilities. This could be reduced by involving more women in their management, or as caretakers, with appropriate incentives to compensate for their time. An alternative or additional modification would be to raise awareness among all community members about the right of girls and women to access the facilities without having to engage in sexual bargaining; in addition, a mechanism for reporting and dealing with complaints should be established.

The possibility of exclusion from water and sanitation projects suggests two ideas for modification. First, where the poorest households cannot afford to pay for access to water and sanitation facilities, a safety-net of some kind could secure them that access, provided that it is designed in a way that does not threaten the sustainability of the project. Second, if community members prevented people from AIDS-affected households from using the facilities, fearing that they would somehow transmit HIV to others, then education work should explain how HIV is transmitted. In other cases of exclusion, the management committee could act to secure access to the facilities.

Education

Education generally reduces susceptibility to HIV and vulnerability to the impacts of AIDS. A girl who has received a basic education is, at least in theory, more able to take charge of her life, earn a living, respond to health-promotion messages, and plan for her future. She is also more able to claim her rights, for example, in terms of access to health care, or securing her inheritance. However, if she is pressured or forced into unprotected sex by male teachers or pupils, her susceptibility to HIV infection is raised. One strategy to reduce this possibility is to raise the awareness of teachers and pupils about pupils' rights, and in particular the rights of girls and women, at the same time as establishing appropriate complaints procedures and disciplinary measures.

Education could have a greater impact on reducing pupils' susceptibility and vulnerability if it helped them to learn important life skills: not only the ability to read and write, but also to reflect on problems, find solutions and make decisions, and acquire practical skills to earn a living. To do this, the content of what is taught, and the training given to teachers, need to be adapted to make education more attractive and useful to pupils.

Education could do more to reduce susceptibility and vulnerability if all children attended school. The exclusion of the poorest or most vulnerable children, and in particular girls, might be tackled by reducing or waiving school fees and reducing the cash costs of attending school (the costs of uniforms, books, and special project payments). More flexible hours might enable children who have competing responsibilities to attend school, and incentives such as providing lunch could also increase the proportion of children who regularly attend school.

In summary, ideas for devising development work which maximises the ways in which it indirectly responds to HIV and AIDS include the following:

- Modify work in all sectors to reduce the likelihood of increasing susceptibility and vulnerability, and to maximise the positive effects.

- Strengthen household safety-nets, through improving incomes and building up household assets by promoting low-risk agriculture and micro-finance initiatives suited to vulnerable households.

Adapting systems

If mainstreaming is to become a standard part of what organisations do, they need to alter the systems and procedures that guide and discipline both the staff and the organisation. Two sets of systems are considered here: those relating to employees, and those concerned with the project cycle.

Employees' roles and responsibilities

Each staff member's responsibility for considering HIV/AIDS can be formalised by including it in all job descriptions, in appraisal mechanisms, and in induction procedures. The wording should ideally arise from the organisation's own mainstreaming process, so using the vocabulary which the organisation has adopted and which makes sense to staff. General references to 'attention to AIDS' are not enough; it would be better to require staff (for example) to be 'alert to, and act upon, the ways in development work can increase or decrease both susceptibility to HIV infection, and vulnerability to the impacts of AIDS'.

Employees' terms and conditions should also include standards of behaviour – for example, regarding honesty and non-discrimination against HIV-infected people – and disciplinary procedures for offences such as corruption and sexual harassment or abuse. For the organisation as a whole, the commitment to respond to HIV/AIDS as a mainstream issue (and perhaps also as an issue requiring specialised AIDS work) should be clearly stated in key documents, such as a mission statement.

The project cycle

If mainstreaming is to become a fundamental feature of the organisation's way of working, it must be incorporated in the project cycle: all the tools and steps from start to finish need to attend to HIV/AIDS and gender, regardless of the sector.

At the needs-assessment stage, staff should learn about the current and likely future impacts of HIV and AIDS, and related issues such as gender inequality, sexual and reproductive health, sexual norms, violence, abuse of alcohol and other drugs, and migration. These can be explored through participatory appraisal methods, such as those described earlier in this chapter in the section about undertaking community research.

At the project-planning stage, staff need to consider those issues, and their links to the project, as described in the preceding section on designing development work which indirectly affects HIV and AIDS. Although one cannot predict the consequences of a project, one can explore possible effects and outcomes with potential participants while designing the project. This should allow the organisation to anticipate and prevent some of the likely problems, including ones which might heighten susceptibility to HIV infection or vulnerability to the impacts of AIDS. In terms of project aims and objectives, it is a good idea to make explicit references to features of the design which are intended, among other things, to enhance the way in which the project works against HIV/AIDS, and to include specific means of monitoring those features.

Concern with the project's effects on susceptibility and vulnerability need to be borne in mind during implementation, and to be included explicitly in monitoring and evaluation measures and in reporting. Moreover, for HIV/AIDS to be successfully mainstreamed in an organisation's systems, monitoring and revision of the adaptations themselves are needed. This would involve checking that users understand the references to the condition, and are able to use them in meaningful ways.

In summary, ideas for adapting systems in order to establish mainstreaming as a standard part of development work include the following:

- Include attention to mainstreaming HIV/AIDS in job descriptions, appraisal mechanisms, and documents concerning the organisation's purpose and approach.

- Deal with issues relating to HIV susceptibility in employees' terms and conditions of employment.

- Incorporate the actions needed to mainstream HIV/AIDS in all stages of the project cycle.

External mainstreaming in development work: a summary

This chapter has presented four steps in external mainstreaming by development agencies, which are summarised in Figure 8.1. It has described how development programmes which build on households' own risk-reduction strategies, such as trying to increase income and build up assets, are likely to be valuable in reducing both susceptibility to HIV and vulnerability to the impacts of AIDS. The chapter has also presented some ideas for mainstreaming HIV/AIDS within the sectors of agriculture, micro-finance, primary health care, water and sanitation, and education.

Figure 8.1 Summary of key steps in the external mainstreaming of HIV/AIDS in development work

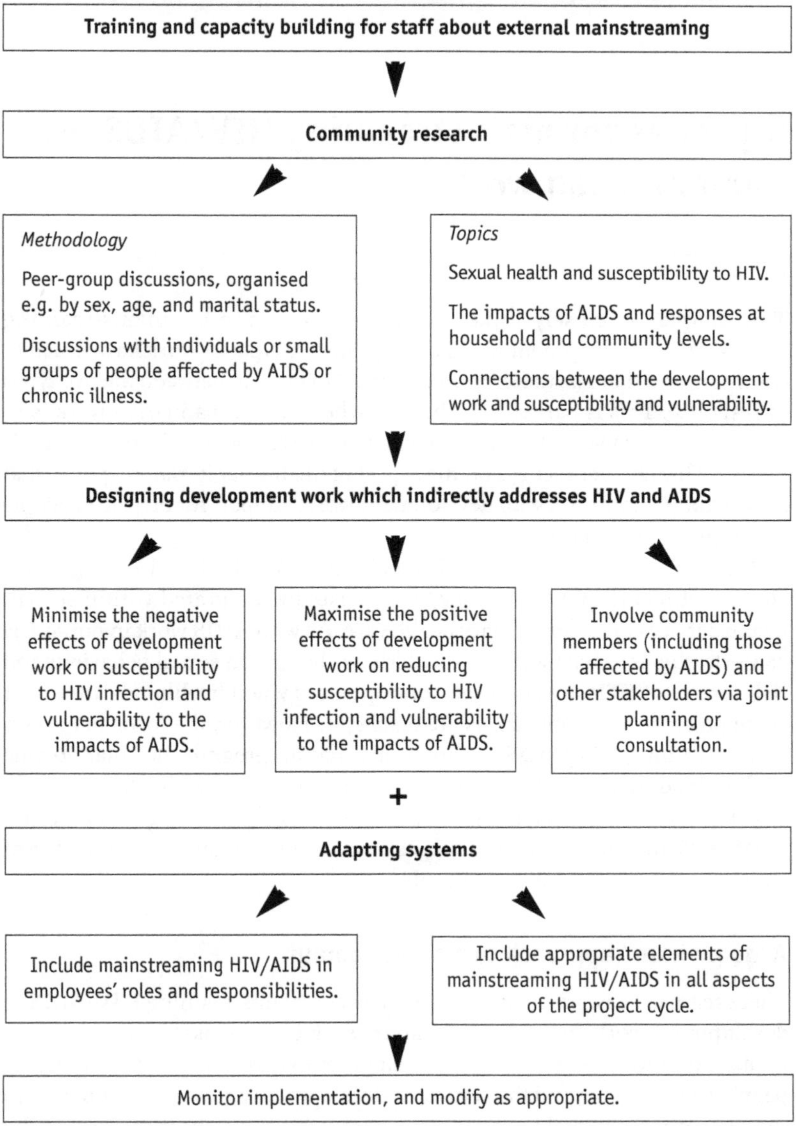

Training and capacity building for staff about external mainstreaming

Community research

Methodology

Peer-group discussions, organised e.g. by sex, age, and marital status.

Discussions with individuals or small groups of people affected by AIDS or chronic illness.

Topics

Sexual health and susceptibility to HIV.

The impacts of AIDS and responses at household and community levels.

Connections between the development work and susceptibility and vulnerability.

Designing development work which indirectly addresses HIV and AIDS

Minimise the negative effects of development work on susceptibility to HIV infection and vulnerability to the impacts of AIDS.

Maximise the positive effects of development work on reducing susceptibility to HIV infection and vulnerability to the impacts of AIDS.

Involve community members (including those affected by AIDS) and other stakeholders via joint planning or consultation.

+

Adapting systems

Include mainstreaming HIV/AIDS in employees' roles and responsibilities.

Include appropriate elements of mainstreaming HIV/AIDS in all aspects of the project cycle.

Monitor implementation, and modify as appropriate.

9 | Ideas for mainstreaming HIV/AIDS in humanitarian work

This chapter is closely linked to the previous one on mainstreaming HIV/AIDS in development work. Clearly, the two types of work have much in common, and there is, therefore, a great deal of overlap between the two types of response. This is particularly the case where the humanitarian work is in response to a slow-onset crisis, and when people are not displaced from their homes. This chapter focuses on the aspect of the humanitarian response that most strongly contrasts with development work: support for displaced people or refugees living in camps.

Many of the papers and policies about HIV/AIDS and emergencies concern direct responses to HIV/AIDS, usually integrated within sexual-health services or wider primary health care. As with AIDS work in non-crisis contexts, this is crucial work, particularly as changes in sexual behaviour and rising rates of STIs are common consequences when livelihoods are under acute pressure and populations are displaced. However, the focus here is on mainstreaming HIV/AIDS in core humanitarian programmes that provide shelter, food, water, and basic health services. Unfortunately, there are very few documented experiences of this, and a large gap between policy and practice. With this in mind, the suggestions in this chapter are ideas (many of which are theoretical) rather than rules.

A 'do no harm' approach to mainstreaming

There seem to be two main differences between mainstreaming HIV/AIDS in development work and in humanitarian work in fast-onset crises involving population movements. First, in development work, most factors affecting people's lives are beyond the control of development agencies. In contrast, in refugee camps, external agencies play a part in deciding where people live; the types of food and non-food items that are mainly available, and who gets what; where people get water from; and the health services on offer. They also influence who gets the limited amount of formal employment that is available, and who benefits from training and education. This also applies, to a lesser extent, in situations where a population has been displaced but has integrated with the host community.

The decisions that agencies make have an impact on all the different kinds of people whom they are aiming to serve. Some of the known negative effects are increased gender inequality, sexual and gender-based violence, sexual abuse, and sexual trading. This justifies the principle that, given agencies' wider field of influence in such contexts, their frame of reference must extend to include these difficult but important issues. The special circumstances tend to shift the mainstreaming agenda away from HIV/AIDS to broader factors such as sexual violence, which demand attention in their own right, in addition to their connection with HIV transmission.

The second difference relates to phases within the humanitarian response. In the later stages, when a situation has stabilised, agencies should be undertaking development work, such as supporting households to develop their livelihoods, to build their assets, and to improve their skills and capacity. An agency which is doing development work in a humanitarian setting can meaningfully mainstream HIV/AIDS, as already discussed in Chapter 8. For example, it can consider how to ensure that its programmes include and serve the development needs of vulnerable households, how to reduce susceptibility to HIV infection through reducing poverty and empowering women, and how to help households to become less vulnerable to the impacts of AIDS. This also applies in slow-onset disasters, when the community has not been displaced.

However, in the early stages of a fast-onset emergency with population displacement, there is the short-term imperative of trying to meet basic needs and to help people to stay alive. While this relief phase lasts, it is probably not meaningful to think of fully mainstreaming HIV/AIDS. Quite aside from the logistical pressures that agencies face at such times, there is also a theoretical reason for this. The idea of mainstreaming HIV/AIDS depends on the ability of development work to address the root causes and consequences of the pandemic; but relief-based humanitarian work which only helps people to survive cannot address the deep development issues that drive HIV and AIDS. It is proposed, then, that in instances where agencies are necessarily focused on helping people to survive rather than to develop, it is more realistic and relevant to focus on a 'do no harm' form of mainstreaming; in other words, trying to ensure that their work does not cause harm by increasing susceptibility to HIV infection. The rationale for prioritising this aspect of mainstreaming is that the work of humanitarian agencies seems to have the greatest influence on susceptibility to HIV infection, particularly in the early stages of the emergency response, and particularly when working in camp situations.

In summary, general ideas for mainstreaming in humanitarian work include the following:

- Use the same principles and approach employed when mainstreaming in development work.
- When humanitarian work is in a relief-focused stage, adopt a limited 'do no harm' form of mainstreaming, centred on minimising unintended negative effects on susceptibility to HIV infection.
- Adopt the full mainstreaming agenda in stable situations in which humanitarian work is moving towards development work.

Training and capacity building

Unlike mainstreaming HIV/AIDS in development work, many of the ideas for mainstreaming in humanitarian work are already present in policies and guidelines, via attention to gender-related concerns and issues of sexual and gender-based violence. Advocacy and training, then, may need to focus less on getting the issue recognised, and more on building commitment and capacity to ensure that practice accords with policy. If senior staff are convinced of the need to do this, then training for other staff can begin. Such training might cover the links between emergencies, gender, and HIV/AIDS; the arguments for mainstreaming; and steps in the mainstreaming process. It could also include refugees' rights and the content of key policies, to ensure that staff understand their duties. This could then lead to considering the practical implications for the humanitarian response, allowing staff to define the next steps in mainstreaming for themselves.

Training and capacity building for field workers will depend on their relationship with the organisation. Where existing employees and partners are involved in the humanitarian response, they could be given basic training in advance; for example, training on gender and emergencies, perhaps associated with courses about the external mainstreaming of HIV/AIDS in development work. The conceptual approach to addressing HIV/AIDS indirectly, and the skills to do so and to carry out community research, apply equally to both situations. For employees recruited for the humanitarian response, rapid induction training is required, which might be facilitated by having simple, pre-prepared training resources.

Ideally every employee in humanitarian work should have a thorough understanding of gender issues and their relationship to HIV/AIDS, and be skilled in researching and devising appropriate responses. However, when under pressure, it may be more realistic to adopt a 'division of labour' strategy, whereby the emphasis of all except basic training is on capacity building for a certain group. These can be characterised as 'software' staff, who concentrate on social aspects of humanitarian work such as community consultation or public-health promotion, working alongside 'hardware' employees who specialise in the technical inputs such as water engineering.

In summary, ideas for training and capacity building for mainstreaming HIV/AIDS in humanitarian work include the following:

- Use existing policies and guidelines within training, to close the gap between policy and practice.

- Expose development staff to ideas about gender, emergencies, and mainstreaming in humanitarian work, perhaps at the same time as training them to mainstream HIV/AIDS in development work.

- Undertake rapid training for new staff recruited for humanitarian work.

- Train all staff in gender issues, but focus further training efforts on certain groups of staff, rather than trying to train everyone equally.

Emergency preparedness

Emergency preparedness is an important means of improving the overall quality of an emergency response, and good practice in this regard has already been mapped and documented. Within that wider task, being prepared for mainstreaming is likely to be critical to attempts to address HIV/AIDS indirectly: an organisation which does not consider mainstreaming issues in advance is highly unlikely to consider them when a crisis strikes.

Training in advance, and having training resources ready for use, are part of being prepared for mainstreaming HIV/AIDS. It may also be worthwhile to identify potential employees in advance, particularly with regard to posts which may be difficult to fill, or in connection with goals such as 'employing more women'. Planning is another element: developing ideas and strategies for how to mainstream HIV/AIDS within the humanitarian response, and how to monitor its effects. This is likely to involve reviewing existing guidelines, making any changes that may be required, and thinking about how to proceed: for example, obtaining additional resources, or prioritising certain aspects, such as phasing from a 'do no harm' approach to full mainstreaming as the response shifts from a relief focus to a development mode. Organisations should also consider in advance the circumstances under which they would or would not become involved in direct AIDS work.

Research is another element of preparedness for mainstreaming HIV/AIDS. Among all the other information which helps to inform the initial humanitarian response, there should, as a minimum, be data on the HIV-prevalence rates in the region, differentiated by sex, age, and location. This information is available from UNAIDS, though it is very incomplete in situations of on-going conflict and disruption. For mainstreaming HIV/AIDS, however, other information is likely to be more useful, such as attitudes and practices concerning gender roles, sexuality, relationships, gender-based violence, and significant cultural differences between different ethnic groups.

Some of this information might be available internally, such as findings from community research as part of development work, while other data might be gathered from local CBOs and NGOs, government ministries, research institutes, and development literature.

Community research

Methods of needs assessment and other forms of research are already presented in agency manuals. The Sphere Project's *Humanitarian Charter and Minimum Standards in Disaster Response* (Sphere Project 2000), for example, does pay attention to gender issues and questions concerning sexual and gender-based violence. Those questions correlate with the 'do no harm' form of mainstreaming, where an agency concentrates on reducing the likelihood that its work will unintentionally increase susceptibility to HIV infection. The Sphere Project also includes standards of good practice for involving women in decision making, and for considering equity and safety.

Research and consultation are central to good practice in humanitarian work, but they may often be neglected, particularly in the early stages of the response when the need to act quickly to 'save lives' takes precedence. However, if consultation can begin at the beginning, rather than after the response has already begun, then the work is likely to be more effective, particularly with regard to gender equality. Some of the researchers should ideally be women, because women and girls in the community are less likely to discuss sensitive problems with male researchers. When the emergency has stabilised, it may be possible to train and involve community members in on-going research and consultation methods. This may be particularly effective if linked to action: for example, women's groups setting up support services for survivors of sexual violence, or, with regard to AIDS work, community-led home-based care programmes.

As with community research as part of development work, all kinds of people need to be involved, including marginalised and particularly vulnerable groups whose ideas and needs are otherwise ignored. It is almost always useful to discuss issues in peer groups, which might be formed on the basis of sex, age, current status (for example, unaccompanied child, or female household head), clan or ethnic group, or any other significant difference within the population. As a minimum, researchers need to listen to men and women separately. In addition they should ideally consult with members of the host community, who are also greatly affected by the crisis and entitled to benefit from the humanitarian response. If researchers are to use community representatives as key informants, women and younger people should be among them.

Designing humanitarian work which indirectly addresses HIV and AIDS

This section reviews ideas for how three standard aspects of a humanitarian response can take account of HIV/AIDS and related issues, mainly focusing on the 'do no harm' approach of minimising increases in susceptibility to HIV infection, along with preventing sexual and gender-based violence. As already stated, however, the ideas concern the extreme situation of refugee camps; it is assumed that in humanitarian work with settled communities, the response is more likely to be closely allied to that already presented in Chapter 8 for mainstreaming in development work.

First, the type and layout of accommodation will affect refugees' susceptibility to HIV infection. Ideally, unrelated families should not have to share the same accommodation; if this is necessary, each family needs as much privacy as possible. Regarding settlement layout, one way to reduce the potential for tension and violence, including sexual violence, is to try to replicate the community's ordinary norms of physical and social accommodation, rather than imposing new systems. Related to this is the idea of grouping households from the same village or location together. Unaccompanied women may be more vulnerable to the risk of rape and may need secure accommodation; the means of achieving this might be based on the community's pre-existing ways of protecting single women such as widows, or on new methods proposed by the women and the wider community: neighbourhood watch groups, for example. Certainly, they must be consulted, and should not be housed in isolated areas, nor grouped together in separate locations.

Second, tap-stands, latrines, and washing facilities should ideally be decentralised, so that each is shared by a number of households, rather than centrally located. Aside from the convenience of having facilities nearby, this means that girls and women do not have to walk long distances to reach them, which may be particularly dangerous at night. When this is not possible, such as during the early stage of the response, organisations should consult women about how to allocate the available latrines: assigning them to a number of families, or designating them as separate facilities for men and women. Where latrines are sited in large groups, for example in public spaces such as market places, those for men and women should be separate, because communal arrangements provide more cover for potential attackers, and increase women's fears. Providing lighting also reduces the risk of attack and lessens fears among users.

Third, in camps and settled communities, there is the issue of distribution systems for food, shelter materials, basic items such as clothing, soap, and cooking utensils, and – depending on circumstances – water and firewood. The goal is for the systems to be fair, so that each individual gets the due ration. Some organisations are already giving all women the right to be registered independently and so receive their allocation in their own right, rather than through their partners. When food is desperately awaited, crowds and violence may stop women and other vulnerable people from getting their rations, or the rations may be taken from them. Organisations can reduce the risk of this through advance planning, security measures, and clear information about entitlements. Another strategy is to involve women in managing the actual distribution, so as to reduce unfair practices which discriminate against women. This should also reduce the incidence of sexual abuse or bartering in connection with distribution. However, this strategy may be counterproductive, because in some cases women appointed to distribute items have become subject to intimidation and attack.

Connected to distribution is the issue of collecting firewood, which can expose girls and women to sexual violence outside camps. Supervised wood-gathering may reduce the risk of attack. Agencies can also influence the amount of fuel required by each household by providing access to mills, or milled cereals, which cook more quickly than whole grain. Fuel-efficient stoves and cooking pots with well-fitting lids can also reduce the number of trips taken to gather fuel, as can solar cooking methods.

Fourth, the ideas presented in Chapter 8 for mainstreaming HIV/AIDS in primary health care can be transferred to the emergency setting. They mainly concern preventing exclusion and discrimination on the basis of HIV/AIDS.

For each of these components of humanitarian work, organisations should follow up their consultation with monitoring as the work is implemented. This monitoring could focus specifically on the groups of people known to be vulnerable, and most likely to be experiencing problems that might otherwise remain hidden. They may include unaccompanied women and girls, women and children who are heading households, and the chronically sick and their carers (and – less clearly associated with AIDS but vulnerable nonetheless – elderly and disabled people). Monitoring needs to include not only the basic function of the service (for example, the quality of the drinking water) but also users' experience, in a wide sense, of the service. This includes being alert to consequences which heighten susceptibility to HIV infection or vulnerability to the impacts of AIDS. Where appropriate, organisations then need to use monitoring data to stimulate action: for example, to discipline agency staff or other personnel such as peacekeeping forces who are abusing their position of power; to increase security patrols in certain places; or to tackle the exclusion of AIDS-affected people from benefiting equally.

Once an emergency has stabilised, and particularly in cases where refugees or displaced people are unlikely to return home for some time, humanitarian agencies may begin to shift to undertaking development work, such as investing in education, skills training, and income-generation activities.

At this point, the approach to mainstreaming merges with that already presented for mainstreaming in development work in the previous chapter.

In summary, ideas concerning designing humanitarian work which indirectly addresses HIV and AIDS include the following:

- Use existing codes and standards which concur with a 'do no harm' approach.
- Mainstream in all sectors, always with attention to gender issues and a special focus on vulnerable individuals and households.
- Monitor work and adapt it as necessary.
- Move to a full agenda for mainstreaming as soon as is practicable.

Adapting systems

As with external mainstreaming in development work, the task is one of institutionalising attention to HIV/AIDS. The same personnel measures apply – incorporating AIDS-related responsibilities in job descriptions and terms of reference, and in induction and training – along with enforcing appropriate terms and conditions. Agencies are increasingly using codes of conduct for humanitarian workers, but these must be accompanied by means of holding staff accountable to beneficiaries, and methods of disciplining individuals who violate the standards. Finally, organisations need to adapt their own systems with regard to the project cycle; existing policies and guidelines provide a good starting place for this.

External mainstreaming in humanitarian work: a summary

This chapter has presented the main ideas for mainstreaming HIV/AIDS in humanitarian programmes, insofar as they differ from the ideas for development work. It has proposed that in stable situations, and where agencies are working in a developmental way with settled communities, they may adapt and use the ideas for mainstreaming HIV/AIDS in development work. However, in emergencies, such as those arising from fast-onset disasters with mass population movements, it may not be practicable to think of fully mainstreaming HIV/AIDS. Instead, during the relief phase, agencies might focus on a 'do no harm' approach to mainstreaming, trying to limit the ways in which their work may increase susceptibility to HIV and encourage gender and sexual violence. In this regard, the chapter has presented ideas concerning the provision of accommodation, water and sanitation facilities, distribution systems, and health care. Figure 9.1 summarises the main components in the form of a flow chart.

Figure 9.1: Summary of key steps in the external mainstreaming of HIV/AIDS in humanitarian work

Training and capacity building for staff about external mainstreaming

Emergency preparedness

Community research for a 'do no harm' approach to mainstreaming

Methodology	*Topics*
Peer-group discussions, organised for example according to sex, age, and current status (e.g. female heads of household).	Sexual health, sexual violence, gender inequality, and susceptibility to HIV.
Discussions with vulnerable individuals, e.g. unaccompanied girls and women.	Consultation about project design in order to minimise those factors.
Ideally, discussions with members of the host community also.	

Adapting systems

Include mainstreaming HIV/AIDS in employees' roles and responsibilities.	Include appropriate elements of mainstreaming HIV/AIDS in all aspects of the project cycle.

Monitor implementation, and modify as appropriate.

Move to full agenda for mainstreaming HIV/AIDS as the situation stabilises and relief work turns towards development work.

10 | Issues and challenges

This chapter brings together some of the main challenges to the prospects for mainstreaming HIV/AIDS, both internally and externally, and in both development and humanitarian work. First, however, it focuses on two general issues: supporting partners to mainstream, and options for organisations in countries with relatively low rates of HIV prevalence.

Supporting partners to mainstream HIV/AIDS

The principles and ideas already presented in this book apply both to large development organisations and to small community-based organisations. For many larger agencies, however, the task may be not only to mainstream HIV/AIDS in their own organisations, and in their programme work, but to encourage their partners also to address the problem indirectly through their core work. However, this can be problematic: how can they best encourage, support, and empower partners to adopt the mainstreaming agenda, rather than imposing it upon them? Some might choose to provide partners with training, technical support, links to specialists, and funding, but leave them to decide whether or not to mainstream HIV/AIDS. Others may attempt to enforce the mainstreaming agenda by imposing funding conditions. In either case, the donor agency needs to be committed to mainstreaming HIV/AIDS, and must itself be trying to mainstream, if it is to be effective in supporting its partners to do the same.

Strategically, if donors are concerned that partners should preserve their effectiveness, and are concerned with the general health of the CBO sector as a part of civil society, they may want to emphasise and prioritise the internal mainstreaming of HIV/AIDS. In doing so, they will need to recognise, and be willing to pay, the internal costs which arise from mainstreaming, such as health care for staff and dependants (perhaps extending to antiretroviral treatment) and temporary cover for absences.

However, it is very difficult for small organisations to predict and budget for these costs, and particularly the direct costs incurred when a member of staff develops AIDS. An organisation employing 1,000 people, with an assumed rate of AIDS cases of two per cent, can budget for the costs of twenty people, and cope with variations around this figure. However, for a CBO with only ten staff and a similar rate of AIDS, one fifth of a person may be expected to have AIDS. Obviously, when a member of staff does fall ill, it will be a whole person rather than a fraction. The CBO could budget on the basis of one fifth each year. However, this would be insufficient if someone did develop AIDS; and, if there were no case of AIDS, many donors would not allow the money to be carried over to the next year. One way to resolve this problem is for donor agencies to encourage their partners to have proper workplace policies and to budget accordingly, but to hold a central fund on which any partner can draw. By budgeting centrally for the total number of people employed by all the partners, the donor agency ought to be able to make appropriate provisions. However, the situation is complicated by the fact that CBOs often receive support from several donors simultaneously.

The other implication for small organisations is that it is all the more important to share knowledge and practices among the staff, in order to minimise disruptions when an employee is absent. Although small organisations may have more fluid work practices and a less rigid division of labour than large agencies, they may be more vulnerable with regard to sickness among people in key posts. For example, there may be only one person with skills in computing or accounting. Clear record keeping and budgeted contingency plans can help to reduce the impact of the absence of such important post-holders.

Experience so far suggests that partners may need more support in external mainstreaming than in internal mainstreaming, particularly in terms of understanding the indirect links between their work and HIV/AIDS, and devising appropriate modifications. Donor organisations could provide additional support beyond training workshops, such as assisting partners in their community research, and in their process of defining and trying out adaptations.

In summary, ideas for agencies which are supporting partners to mainstream HIV/AIDS include the following.

- Ensure that your agency is committed to mainstreaming, and understands it, before attempting to influence partners.
- Devise and fund an appropriate mix of on-going support and persuasion.
- Help partners to budget for the internal costs of treatment for HIV and AIDS.
- Recognise that internal and external mainstreaming may mean higher costs, both financial and non-financial.

Mainstreaming HIV/AIDS where HIV-prevalence rates are low

This book is mainly based on experiences in countries in Southern and Eastern Africa, where the rates of HIV prevalence are high, and the impacts of generalised HIV epidemics are already very evident. But how should agencies respond to the mainstreaming agenda in circumstances where HIV-prevalence rates are low? The following ideas are theoretical; they fall into three categories.

One option is to do nothing, which has the merit of being cost-free, and gives organisations the opportunity to wait for mainstreaming lessons to emerge as other agencies experiment. However, in the mean time, the agency gains nothing, loses the opportunity to act in advance of rising rates of HIV infection, and may incur higher costs in the long term.

A second option is to adopt the same mainstreaming processes as described in this section of the book, but at a lower level of intensity. This approach is similar to disaster preparedness, in the sense of preparing both employees and the organisation for the possibility of rising HIV prevalence and its associated risks and consequences. In large organisations with programmes around the world, the strategy also means that all programmes are on an equal footing, and are all ready and able to respond. The disadvantage of this approach is that it may be very difficult to motivate people to invest in mainstreaming where HIV rates are low. This is true for internal mainstreaming, but even more so for external mainstreaming, where none of the impacts of AIDS will be evident. Both employees and community members will find it difficult to appreciate the probable consequences of AIDS and their implications for development or humanitarian work.

A third option is to apply mainstreaming processes to attend to issues related to HIV/AIDS, such as gender inequality, and the need to strengthen household safety-nets. This has the advantage that, rather than attempting to impose an agenda on employees and community members who have few concerns about HIV/AIDS, organisations can respond to issues which are of concern, and which require attention regardless of whether or not infection rates rise. It has the disadvantage that additional work specific to AIDS would be necessary if HIV rates were to rise.

As the first option requires no further explanation, and the second is based on all that has come before – i.e. mainstreaming HIV/AIDS – this section outlines some ideas for the third option.

Internal mainstreaming of AIDS-related issues in low-prevalence settings

With regard to internal mainstreaming, measures to support staff could simply focus on wider health issues, including STIs (which include HIV), because it is beneficial for employees and the organisation alike for staff to be motivated to look after their physical and mental health. Staff could jointly consider their organisational culture to see if some elements – such as the use and abuse of alcohol at workshops, or at the end of the week – might usefully be changed. Non-health topics which might be of interest to staff include financial management, communication skills, and conflict resolution. All of these might have current appeal and relevance, but with indirect benefits in terms of reducing susceptibility to STIs, including HIV infection, and vulnerability to external shocks, including AIDS.

With regard to workplace policies, gender equality is probably the most likely topic to seem relevant to staff and to meet the organisation's needs. A similar mainstreaming process, based on the same broad principles, could then be applied: acknowledging the issue through research, then learning through workshops before devising a policy. Ideally the non-discrimination section of any policy could also cover HIV/AIDS (along with other factors such as age, ethnicity, and disability). The process and outcome would be useful to the organisation in terms of formulating its values with regard to gender, and agreeing on measures to promote equality and to act against discrimination.

In terms of modifying how the organisation functions, several of the measures suggested for mainstreaming HIV/AIDS internally would be beneficial to organisations unaffected by AIDS. For example, many organisations do not have effective systems for coping with expected absences of staff (such as maternity leave), let alone unexpected staff shortages caused by illness, or sudden departures when an employee leaves without giving notice. Even when a member of staff gives notice, there is commonly a period when other employees have to cover the post while the recruitment process goes on, sometimes slowly and ineffectively. Moreover, where people tend to work independently and not share work tasks, the organisational culture may be unsupportive and isolating. A lack of information about staff leave and the implementation of personnel policies may also add to inefficiency, or unfair treatment of staff. Setting up systems to gather such data would, in time, allow management to analyse staff costs and options with greater accuracy. Overall, addressing any or all of these issues would help an organisation to function, and reduce its vulnerability to impacts as and when AIDS strikes its employees and their families.

External mainstreaming of AIDS-related issues in low-prevalence settings

The idea of mainstreaming HIV/AIDS is based on the notion that development and humanitarian work, when well done, is indirectly acting against HIV and AIDS. In that sense, all that the agencies need to do is to continue doing their work. However, as Chapter 4 explained, development and humanitarian work may, without meaning to, increase susceptibility and vulnerability. This book has argued that mainstreaming can reduce that tendency, while also strengthening the ways in which the work acts to reduce susceptibility and vulnerability.

This argument is valid even if HIV is not present, because the underlying causes, such as gender inequality and poverty, remain. In other words, work which does not take account of the factors of gender inequality and poverty may be working with, rather than against, them. While poverty reduction is assumed to be to be at the heart of development and humanitarian work, this does not mean that the work is always in the best interests of poor people. Furthermore, gender issues are often ignored and made worse by development and humanitarian work. In situations where HIV prevalence is low, or where AIDS is not recognised as an issue, organisations could decide to review their work in order to make it more poverty-focused and 'pro-poor'. This might result, for example, in refocusing agricultural extension work towards supporting subsistence farmers who have few resources, with the aim of strengthening their household safety-nets and so reducing their vulnerability to shocks, including AIDS. Alternatively, or at the same time, organisations could adopt a process of gender mainstreaming. This might result, for example, in agricultural extension work being redesigned to include women farmers, and to respond to their needs more effectively.

It is important to note, however, that neither of these processes is the same as mainstreaming HIV/AIDS. While attending to the effects of the pandemic requires knowledge of, and attention to, issues of gender and poverty, there are core aspects of mainstreaming HIV/AIDS which would not be dealt with through becoming more poverty-focused or through mainstreaming gender equality. These aspects are concerned with the impacts of AIDS, now and in the future, and both within organisations and among community members. Hence, an organisation which attends to poverty or gender in a low-HIV setting would still need to attend to mainstreaming HIV/AIDS if prevalence rose among the general population. However, the organisation's work in the low-prevalence phase would have begun to fight HIV and AIDS before they became significant, so laying useful foundations for the subsequent process of mainstreaming HIV/AIDS.

Within development and humanitarian work, certain types of programme may be particularly relevant to acting against AIDS in advance of rising HIV-prevalence. At the general level, this includes all efforts to empower women, to address sexual and gender-based violence, and to improve the status of women and girls. A more specific route is sexual-health and reproductive-health programmes, and in particular efforts to reduce unwanted pregnancies, and to promote biomedical treatment of STIs. It also includes all poverty-focused efforts to support livelihood security, and in particular to help poor households to raise their incomes and to build up their assets, so becoming less poor and less vulnerable to the impacts of external shocks.

Organisations could also aim to help people to build up their productive assets, for instance by planting fruit trees or cash crops which take time to establish but then provide a reliable harvest, with relatively low labour requirements. A less obvious route involves improving the productive use of income, aimed at enabling men and women to analyse their expenditure and to realise more of the poverty-alleviating potential of their income.

In terms of strategy, and regardless of sector, work which helps to build civil society through empowering community organisations seems to result in more robust communities which are better able to meet their needs and to tackle new challenges. Any inclusive development and humanitarian work which helps to build civil society is a force against poverty and gender inequality, and hence, indirectly, it works against HIV and AIDS.

Finally, although this section concerns options for responding to the agenda for mainstreaming HIV/AIDS in low-prevalence settings, it is important to remember the option of AIDS work. In situations where HIV infection is still concentrated among 'high-risk' population sub-groups, there is a very important opportunity to try to reduce the rate of new infections among those groups, and to prevent HIV from crossing over to the broader population. Indeed, in more than twenty years of AIDS-prevention work, the notable successes have been achieved through focused and empowering work with population sub-groups, before HIV infection has spread to the general population. An organisation is more likely to achieve significant impacts by investing in needle-exchange programmes for injecting drug-users, or in comprehensive programmes for concentrated groups of commercial sex workers, than by undertaking HIV-prevention work for a whole population. Furthermore, the strategy of STI treatment as a means of reducing the rate of new HIV infections is more effective when focused on members of 'high-risk' groups, before HIV infection becomes generalised, because they are likely to transmit HIV to greater numbers of people (Barnett and Whiteside 2002:329).

Challenges to mainstreaming

This section considers the main challenges that are faced by supporters of mainstreaming HIV/AIDS. It begins by identifying the main brakes on starting the mainstreaming process, and then discusses some of the challenges within the process.

Brakes on getting started

Advocates of mainstreaming HIV/AIDS face many problems in their efforts to persuade organisations to accept the argument for mainstreaming, and to commit themselves to action.

Lack of clarity over the meaning of mainstreaming

The term 'mainstreaming HIV/AIDS' is used to mean several different things, and often to mean nothing very specific, which makes it difficult for everyone, from donors and governments to NGOs and CBOs, to talk to each other about the issue. It also makes the whole topic confusing and contradictory, which may deter some people from thinking about the notion of mainstreaming HIV/AIDS. Moreover, the confusion over terminology may undermine implementation, if organisations embark on their mainstreaming process without a common sense among employees of what they are trying to achieve. All of this may add up to a situation in which the term 'mainstreaming' becomes degraded or discarded, along with the concepts and aims behind it. More positively, however, a growing number of agencies and governments are beginning to understand and implement mainstreaming as it is presented in this book; as more join them, generating further debate and experience, greater clarity may be achieved.

Mainstreaming is complex to explain and difficult to promote

Mainstreaming HIV/AIDS is a difficult concept to promote, particularly in comparison with the task of advocating for direct AIDS work. To begin with, mainstreaming is not an obvious strategy; it requires people to think in a new way, and the arguments behind it are rather complex. This means that advocacy for mainstreaming HIV/AIDS involves explaining mainstreaming; and even if advocates' explanations are simple but thorough, their audiences may need time before they understand the concept, or they may misunderstand it. For example, in the response to the recent food crisis in Southern Africa, mainstreaming HIV/AIDS became understood as ensuring that food aid reached 'AIDS-affected' households. This led to the risk that indicators of being 'AIDS-affected', such as households with a member with chronic illness, could be used to target food aid, rather than using indicators of food insecurity or of standard wealth criteria (Harvey 2004:176).

A further problem is that the outcomes of mainstreaming HIV/AIDS are not, by its nature, very visible, so they may not be easily captured and communicated, as part of advocacy for mainstreaming, in words or pictures. Of course, advocacy is further challenged by the current lack of experience in mainstreaming, and by the absence of hard evidence that supporters of mainstreaming can present in support of their arguments.

To meet this challenge, advocates for mainstreaming need to find ways of presenting the logic of the concept, and illustrating the process and its outcomes, in more easily understood ways. The concept will always be more complex than, say, the straightforward case that HIV-positive people have a right to treatment, but it should be possible to improve the way in which the case for mainstreaming is phrased and presented. The case for mainstreaming could also be simplified by compromising; for example, presenting mainstreaming as being mainly about reducing vulnerability, so setting aside the whole aspect of susceptibility, and the unintended negative effects which development and humanitarian work may have on both aspects.

In addition to finding better ways to communicate about mainstreaming, advocates need more experience to which to refer, in order to demonstrate that mainstreaming can enhance the contribution made by development and humanitarian work to the overall response to HIV/AIDS. This requires agencies not only to experiment with implementing mainstreaming, but to monitor and evaluate their work, to document it thoroughly, and to share their experiences. These requirements present further challenges, which are considered later in this chapter.

Mainstreaming lacks a group of supporters

Another brake on mainstreaming HIV/AIDS is that it does not have a natural group of advocates. AIDS-related advocacy is mainly done by groups of people who are HIV-positive and are fighting for their rights to be protected – and fighting in particular for access to treatment. For AIDS activists, these immediate and important issues understandably predominate. Advocacy for mainstreaming HIV/AIDS requires a longer and broader perspective, and a more complex analysis; it seems more likely to emerge from development agencies and other institutions than from the grassroots. Indeed, as the impacts of AIDS on organisations, communities, and development work are becoming more obvious in highly affected regions, interest in mainstreaming HIV/AIDS is also growing. Although the distinctive strategies of mainstreaming HIV/AIDS and integrating AIDS work are usually mixed up, growing interest among donors, planners, and development agencies presents an opportunity to be exploited by advocates of mainstreaming.

Organisations lack the resources to undertake mainstreaming

While larger development organisations which are determined to mainstream should be able to find the funds from within to do so, small organisations are more likely to depend on funds from outside. However, the combination of problems described above means that mainstreaming is not a high priority for donors. They are much more willing to provide funds for HIV-prevention programmes, or for programmes supporting orphans or providing care. Even donors that seek to fund projects of 'impact mitigation' generally prefer such work to be clearly designed to deliver benefits to people directly affected by AIDS, rather than taking the broader approach of adapting existing development work.

Another possible challenge is that donors may wrongly ascribe new budget lines and higher core costs resulting from mainstreaming to bad management, and choose to invest in organisations which appear to offer 'better value'. An organisation might incur higher costs if it upgrades the treatments available to employees who are HIV-positive, while the benefits – in terms of continuity, staff morale, and the reputation of the organisation – are not visible in the accounts. This implies that organisations need to explain the rationale, costs, and benefits of mainstreaming clearly to their donors, and to use their experiences to support advocacy for mainstreaming within the wider development community.

Even where an organisation does not need substantial funds to mainstream, it may need technical support. As the idea of mainstreaming gains more prominence, and as people become more aware of the challenges that HIV/AIDS is presenting to their work and their organisations, there is more interest in the concept. However, along with confusion over what main-streaming means, there is uncertainty about what it is supposed to achieve, and how to do it. A manager who is interested in mainstreaming and who seeks support will find a limited range of publications, and, with the exception of institutional audits, almost no organisations able to offer practical and experience-based technical support. This is not to say that such support cannot emerge – there are organisations with the relevant skills to apply themselves to mainstreaming – but simply that, as yet, they are not numerous.

Short-term survival versus long-term strategy

One of the constraints faced by HIV-prevention programmes is that for poor people the immediate concern of surviving today displaces consideration of possible problems in the future. Women and men who have to live from day to day do not typically invest much time in constructing long-term plans. When seeking to mainstream HIV/AIDS, donor-dependent NGOs and CBOs may similarly prioritise immediate issues – their own survival, in the sense of getting another grant – at the expense of long-term planning. Many 'partnerships' have a lifespan of only a few years, linked to a project grant, and few donor agencies are willing to commit their resources to long-term partnerships.

However, while mainstreaming may not be immediately attractive to organisations unable to afford the luxury of long-term planning, it might become more appealing if they received sufficient support. NGOs and CBOs may be particularly open to the idea of mainstreaming HIV/AIDS internally if they are already feeling the impacts of AIDS, and their sense of 'needing to do something' is growing. Managers may be attracted to the idea that mainstreaming HIV/AIDS can help their organisations to survive AIDS by acting in advance to avoid financial and operational crises. Another possible appeal of mainstreaming is that it may, in time, improve organisations' ability to secure funds from donors, if they can demonstrate that they are prepared for the problem, and that their work will respond to the challenges that it presents.

Challenges within mainstreaming

Organisations attempting to mainstream HIV/AIDS are likely to face many challenges. This section features three particular issues: the lack of complementary partners with whom to make links; the problem of developing effective monitoring and evaluation for mainstreaming; and the need to develop modes for shared learning and networking.

Lack of complementary partners

External mainstreaming means that development and humanitarian organisations should first adapt their core work, rather than beginning with AIDS projects, and then form complementary partnerships with specialist organisations which are dealing with AIDS directly. However, in practice those specialist organisations may not exist, or they may not cover all aspects of AIDS work, or they may be unable to extend themselves to form meaningful partnerships. In such a situation, a small organisation which had intended to mainstream HIV/AIDS might, realistically, face two options: continue with mainstreaming and ignore the need for AIDS work, or abandon mainstreaming and embark on AIDS work. If it had sufficient capacity, it could attempt to undertake both strategies, but at some risk to the quality of both initiatives. A larger organisation with more capacity might be more able to adopt both strategies, and have the additional option of funding and supporting one or more other organisations to begin AIDS work. Each would have to make its own decision, according to its circumstances. This is to acknowledge, however, that the theoretical ideal of focusing on mainstreaming HIV/AIDS and then forming complementary partnerships may not be practical in many situations, and that, given the strong desire to do AIDS work, many organisations may still prioritise their direct response to AIDS over the strategy of mainstreaming.

Monitoring and evaluation

Monitoring and evaluation is a notoriously weak component of much development work, and mainstreaming HIV/AIDS is, so far, no exception. However, monitoring and evaluation are critical for learning about what is effective, for ensuring that modifications resulting from mainstreaming do not do more harm than good, and for assessing the impact of mainstreaming HIV/AIDS. Advocacy for mainstreaming also needs documented examples of its positive effects; the theoretical arguments in this book need to be supported by data from actual experiences.

Suitable means of measuring progress in terms of process, outcomes, and impact need to be generated by practitioners, to fit the work that they are doing and the things that they are trying to achieve. However, it is possible to outline some ideas here. For example, all types of mainstreaming involve training and capacity building, so an indicator of progress is the fact that a workshop has happened. But organising a workshop is not the same as building capacity; receiving feedback from participants that they enjoyed the workshop is not the same as demonstrating benefit in terms of outcomes of improved knowledge, skills, confidence, or motivation. Workshops which fail to achieve these outcomes waste precious resources and will undermine the mainstreaming process. Preliminary and follow-up workshop questionnaires are a quick and low-cost way of approximately assessing outcomes. They also help to focus managers' and trainers' minds on defining the aims of the workshop. Crucially, the results of workshop evaluations can help to improve future workshops on the same topic, and reveal outstanding issues that need attention. Trainers' observations from a workshop should also be instructive, but it should be remembered that they are personal and may not be reliable, in the sense that trainers may have a vested interest in portraying the process as successful.

Monitoring and evaluation needs not only to seek and record indicators of process and outcomes, but also to assess impact. For example, imagine that a workshop about modifying an agricultural project has outcomes in terms of agreed modifications, including ensuring that vulnerable young people are included in agricultural training and that they use inputs offered by extension workers. The workshop participants agree on a single indicator to capture this: the percentage of heads of household (or acting heads of household, caring for bedridden elders) aged under 25 who are in receipt of loans of rabbits. In order to track this indicator, they agree that extension agents should record who receives livestock loans, noting the age and sex of the head of household, or acting head. They set the target that the vulnerable young people should form 20 per cent of the total recipients within two years, and that at least 50 per cent of those receiving livestock loans should be female. Over time, the indicator will allow project staff to see whether the modification is implemented, and to what extent against the target.

However, staff will also need to track the impact and sustainability of the measure. They could use quantitative methods, such as tracking changes in the young people's ownership of assets, but that would be very time-consuming. Qualitative assessments in the form of young people's personal reports may be more feasible and sufficient. Another measure would be to track the rate of loan default among various groups within the project. This would reveal if the modification had altered the cost-effectiveness of the project, and provide warning of any threat to sustainability, or a need to change procedures. For example, if the young people had a very high default rate, staff might need to reconsider whether or not the modification of targeting young people with livestock loans is sustainable. Alternatively, if their rate of loan default is lower than average, this might suggest that they could form a greater proportion of the overall total.

With regard to internal mainstreaming, staff attitudes and practices – for example, concerning condoms, counselling, alcohol use, and sexual relationships with community members – could be tracked by means of an anonymous questionnaire, administered once a year. Numbers of days' absence could be recorded by category, such as sickness, sickness of a dependant, compassionate leave, funeral, or holiday. This information could be presented in the form of averages, or in large organisations as averages for different types of worker, categorised for instance by sex or by grade; recording and comparing it year by year would help to update predictions of the impacts of AIDS on the organisation (**Unit 5** of *AIDS on the Agenda* provides some more ideas; it may be downloaded from http://www.oxfam. org.uk /what_we_do/issues/hivaids/aidsagenda.htm).

One critical aspect of assessing internal mainstreaming is the need to maintain confidentiality. Health clinics can use codes rather than names to protect the identity of those who are claiming HIV-related treatment, but in small organisations it would be intrusive to use the number of claimants as an indicator of the success of a workplace policy. Instead, financial impacts might be monitored through the average medical cost per employee, or medical or insurance costs could be calculated and tracked as a percentage of the overall expenditure on salaries.

Overall, an organisation's monitoring and evaluation measures need to be realistic, in two senses. First, the expectations of mainstreaming (or, indeed, of direct AIDS work) must be feasible and measurable. The familiar project goal of 'minimising HIV transmission' fulfils neither of those criteria. Expecting a partner agency to mainstream HIV/AIDS and requiring the process to have an impact on its work within the final year of funding is similarly unrealistic. Second, very complex methods of monitoring progress and measuring impact may be too expensive and time-consuming to be justifiable. Reasonable methods do require time and commitment, but it may be necessary to rely on imperfect indicators to prevent demands from becoming excessive. Finally, it is important to note that monitoring and evaluation of mainstreaming HIV/AIDS needs to build on existing systems, as part of ordinary systems of data collection and analysis. Special measures are required until mainstreaming ceases to be a special project and has become a standard part of the organisation's work.

Limited means of shared learning

Once organisations can, by virtue of their monitoring and evaluation, confidently identify their successes and failures, they must share their experiences if they are to learn from each other. At present organisations lack specific means for exchanging lessons from mainstreaming HIV/AIDS. To date, efforts to share ideas about mainstreaming have mainly been appended to modes of sharing which are focused on AIDS work, such as satellite sessions at HIV/AIDS conferences, and short articles in newsletters about HIV/AIDS. However, these modes of information exchange, focused on AIDS work, are unlikely to encourage or accommodate increasing levels of dialogue about mainstreaming HIV/AIDS, given the continued need for communication on the many aspects of direct responses to AIDS. Moreover, the mainstreaming agenda needs to draw in people from outside the community of AIDS experts and AIDS activists. While those people may be involved in mainstreaming, the learning process will be based on the experiences of professionals and practitioners from ordinary development and humanitarian work.

For proponents of mainstreaming, there appear to be three reinforcing strategies to follow. First, to continue to broaden the AIDS agenda to include mainstreaming HIV/AIDS, using existing publications and forums. Second, to advocate mainstreaming HIV/AIDS through existing modes of information exchange for wider development work, such as generic or sector-specific conferences, workshops, journals, and newsletters. This might be done most effectively by development professionals, rather than by AIDS specialists. Third, to develop new means of learning and sharing about mainstreaming HIV/AIDS: for example, local workshops or networks.

Summary

This chapter has presented some of the issues and challenges inherent in the concept of mainstreaming HIV/AIDS. Overall, Part 2 of the book has aimed to bring together all the experiences and ideas from the case studies and the literature that were reviewed for *AIDS on the Agenda*, in order to present ideas for mainstreaming HIV/AIDS internally and externally. It has presented some common-sense principles which have much in common with general good practice in development.

- Involve staff and beneficiaries.
- Listen to the most vulnerable people.
- Learn from the process, including the mistakes.
- Pay attention to policy and practice.
- Monitor and evaluate.

At the heart of all this is the idea that mainstreaming HIV/AIDS can result in practical changes which make practical differences, and that those differences can help organisations to function effectively, and to work indirectly against the pandemic, despite the impacts of AIDS on their staff and on community members.

The ideas proposed here have covered a full mainstreaming process, which might be replicated among many field offices, or among organisations and their partners. Mainstreaming HIV/AIDS is not, however, an 'all or nothing' process. Mainstreaming internally but not externally is better than not mainstreaming at all. Providing staff with condoms but not voluntary counselling and HIV testing is better than nothing. The comprehensive approach described here – predicting impact, building capacity, fully supporting staff, establishing a workplace policy, changing personnel and financial procedures, conducting community research, modifying programmes, building preparedness, and adapting systems – may be desirable but difficult. Every organisation considering mainstreaming HIV/AIDS needs to determine its own priorities, and the extent to which it will embrace the whole process, as illustrated in Table 6.2. Similarly, every organisation needs to make strategic decisions about the relative emphasis to place on mainstreaming HIV/AIDS in its ordinary work and on doing direct AIDS work.

11 | Conclusion

In June 2001 the United Nations held a General Assembly Special Session devoted to HIV/AIDS, which resulted in a Declaration of Commitment. Among many other commitments, 180 signatory nations agreed by 2003 to

> ...have in place strategies, policies and programmes that identify and begin to address those factors that make individuals particularly vulnerable to HIV infection, including underdevelopment, economic insecurity, poverty, lack of empowerment of women, lack of education, social exclusion, illiteracy, discrimination, lack of information and/or commodities for self-protection, all types of sexual exploitation of women, girls and boys, including for commercial reasons.
> (UNAIDS 2002:22)

This book, in essence, has not argued that the factors listed in the UN Declaration should be addressed in order to respond to AIDS; instead it has argued that development work to address those factors is vital in its own right, and needs to be relevant to the context of AIDS. In highly affected nations, development and humanitarian organisations are trying to tackle inequality and poverty while AIDS relentlessly compounds and deepens those problems. This book has proposed that those organisations should adopt the following measures:

- Use internal mainstreaming of HIV/AIDS to reduce and cope with the impacts of AIDS, and so continue with their work to tackle inequality and poverty, despite the effects of AIDS on their employees and on their functioning.

- Mainstream HIV/AIDS externally in order to ensure that their programme work is responsive to the changes created by AIDS, and contributes indirectly to the fight against HIV and AIDS.

Fundamentally, the book has presented an additional strategy to that of responding to AIDS directly through AIDS work: it has proposed that 'mainstreaming' should be added to the menu of possible responses – a menu which is, at present, dominated by forms of direct AIDS work. This additional strategy is needed because AIDS work, while it is crucial, is not enough: HIV-prevention work cannot address the underlying causes of susceptibility to HIV infection, and care and treatment of people living with AIDS cannot tackle vulnerability to the consequences of AIDS, particularly among the not-yet-affected. And if, as this book has argued, HIV/AIDS is an endemic problem with no obvious solution, then long-term developmental responses of coping and adapting are needed, rather than a short-term focus on 'stopping AIDS'.

Furthermore, development work with HIV/AIDS mainstreamed in it may sometimes be more appropriate than specialised AIDS work targeted at AIDS-affected households. For example, in countries where there are low levels of school enrolment, it may be more cost-effective, and more equitable, to invest in improving the education system itself, for the benefit of *all* children, including those who are vulnerable, rather than devoting resources to campaigns to enrol AIDS orphans. And savings and credit schemes designed to help poor households to improve their livelihood security may be more sustainable, and yield greater benefits, than schemes which exclusively serve people who know that they are HIV-positive. Of course, in an ideal world, everyone would have access to good-quality services, which would include special measures for people affected by AIDS, as necessary. In the real world, politicians, planners, and development professionals are faced with difficult choices. This book has argued that continuing with development and humanitarian work, but with HIV/AIDS mainstreamed in it, is the most effective course of action for organisations which cannot realistically both mainstream HIV/AIDS and do AIDS work.

However, the book has not suggested that the strategy of mainstreaming HIV/AIDS should replace that of responding directly through AIDS work; both strategies are needed, and they complement each other. Some organisations, in particular the larger and relatively well-resourced ones, may have the capacity to adopt both strategies. Others will not be able to manage that, and so will face a choice: whether to focus on AIDS work or on external mainstreaming of HIV/AIDS. This book argues that all organisations should consider undertaking internal mainstreaming; but it is hoped that, by presenting the case for external mainstreaming, it will, at least, convince them that AIDS work is not the only option for responding to AIDS through programme work. The limited experience to date suggests that organisations are unlikely to undertake 'pure' mainstreaming, because of the strength of the desire to do at least some AIDS work.

Although this book has focused on the idea of mainstreaming HIV/AIDS at the local level, through the work of NGOs, CBOs, and local government, the concept of mainstreaming applies equally to national and international policies. Collins and Rau (2000:56) argue that every level of development work has a role to play:

> ...mainstreaming implies training extension workers to recognise signs of agricultural stress due to labour shortages or asset constraints. Mainstreaming stimulates agricultural planners to promote labour-saving crops or labour-sharing systems. It should encourage agricultural and finance ministers and banks to loosen credit, increase farm prices, and reintroduce subsidies on basic foodstuffs. Mainstreaming involves doing— or doing better—what one is supposed to be doing anyway.

Prospects for mainstreaming HIV/AIDS

It is true that there are many barriers which hinder the mainstreaming of HIV/AIDS; but this section presents a few trends which indicate more optimistic prospects for the mainstreaming agenda.

First, some organisations are aware that direct AIDS work is a worthwhile but inadequate response. Their behaviour-change programmes are not potent enough to stop girls and women from trading sex for favours, or to empower them to insist on safer sex, nor to persuade poor men that they should prioritise their future health above their present pleasures. And organisations which support people living with AIDS find that they can help individuals to accept and manage their HIV status, but cannot undertake the development programmes that might lift their households from poverty, and break the reinforcing cycle of the causes and consequences of AIDS. Although AIDS work is seen to be the default response, there is a growing realisation among organisations of all sizes that the complexity of the problem demands a wider range of responses. As a result, the idea of mainstreaming HIV/AIDS is now attracting attention and interest.

A second factor which may advance mainstreaming is that in highly affected countries the impacts of AIDS on organisations and communities are becoming more obvious and harder to ignore. Sick employees, vacant posts, low morale, and rising health-care costs all illustrate the need for the internal mainstreaming of HIV/AIDS. The business sector has more experience in internal mainstreaming than the not-for-profit sector, partly because it is motivated more by self-interest and the need to protect profit margins. However, NGOs, like commercial companies, wish to survive, and are beginning to recognise the need to protect themselves from AIDS, and to take action to preserve their ability to function effectively despite the pandemic.

Similarly, external mainstreaming is likely to be stimulated when organisations experience the impacts of AIDS on their work – impacts such as low levels of participation, and failing development projects. The way in which organisations, employees, and community members are experiencing the impacts of AIDS may also help people to embrace the idea of mainstreaming.

Third, there are some aspects of mainstreaming which may make it a more attractive and viable prospect than the proposition that all sectors should engage in AIDS work. Fundamentally, mainstreaming does not ask all organisations and ministries and employees to step outside their own sectors and become AIDS workers, or AIDS educators, or AIDS activists. Instead it proposes that they should extend their existing professional expertise by learning ways to take account of gender, HIV/AIDS, and sexual health. In addition, the mainstreaming process does not require community members to prioritise HIV/AIDS as a problem, and it does not require organisations to impose an agenda of AIDS work. Both parties can still focus on community priorities, but with concerns about susceptibility to HIV infection and vulnerability to the impacts of AIDS built into the project as appropriate.

A fourth reason for optimism about the prospects for mainstreaming is that it is beginning to happen: books such as this are part of a growing movement concerned with learning about mainstreaming HIV/AIDS and developing good practice. For example, the British government's Department for International Development is investing in promoting mainstreaming through its bilateral aid programme.

In conclusion, this book argues that mainstreaming HIV/AIDS internally and externally is both necessary and possible. Readers may challenge the argument for mainstreaming, but perhaps this book will further stimulate and contribute to the debate about expanding the response to AIDS. However, the only way to test the book's assertion that mainstreaming can maximise the way in which development and humanitarian programmes work indirectly against HIV and AIDS is through experiment and practice. HIV and AIDS have radically changed the context of development and humanitarian work, and now development and humanitarian work needs to change accordingly.

Appendix 1 | Basic information about HIV and AIDS

Transmission of HIV

The letters HIV stand for Human Immunodeficiency Virus. This is the virus that causes AIDS, the Acquired Immune Deficiency Syndrome. HIV can be transmitted (passed) from one person to another in semen, vaginal fluids, blood, and breast milk. This results in four main ways of spreading it – known as *modes of transmission* – as summarised below.

Table A1 Modes of HIV transmission

Mode of transmission	Notes	Ways to reduce the likelihood of HIV transmission
Sexual intercourse	Transmission of HIV is more likely where the skin is broken, e.g. due to anal sex, rough or violent sex, or the presence of a sexually transmitted infection.	Correct use of condoms. Treatment of sexually transmitted infections.
Unsafe medical procedures	These include using instruments such as needles and scalpels that have not been adequately disinfected or sterilised; using HIV-contaminated blood in transfusions; using HIV-contaminated organs in transplants; and exposing open wounds to HIV-contaminated blood.	Disinfecting or sterilising all equipment. Careful recruitment of blood donors. Screening donated blood for HIV. Use of protective clothing or equipment such as gloves.
Other unsafe practices	E.g. circumcision; decorating the body with markings such as tattoos or scars; and injecting drugs.	Disinfecting or sterilising all equipment, or not sharing equipment.
Mother to child	HIV is transmitted from HIV-positive women to their babies in a quarter to a third of cases, either during pregnancy, or at birth, or through breast feeding.	Giving antiretroviral therapies to the mother and her baby. Delivering the baby by caesarean section. Feeding the baby on formula milk.

It is important to note that the likelihood of HIV transmission varies according to circumstances. For example, individuals are more susceptible to a range of infections, including HIV, if they are malnourished, have other infections, or are generally in poor health. This means that different people engaging in the same type of sexual behaviour may have very different chances of becoming infected with HIV, according to their individual health status. The likelihood of HIV being transmitted also varies according to the type of HIV: some sub-types are more easily acquired than others.

Progress from HIV infection to AIDS

Progression from HIV infection to AIDS is commonly thought of in terms of four stages, as summarised below:

Stages of HIV infection

Stage 1:   Initial infection with HIV, when individuals are particularly infectious, and often have an illness resembling influenza.

Stage 2:   The stage when individuals have no symptoms of HIV infection, except perhaps swollen glands, although they are infectious. HIV is, however, attacking and weakening their immune systems.

Stage 3:   The stage when symptoms of HIV infection are present in the form of opportunistic infections and cancers that the immune system would normally prevent. Periods of ill health can be interspersed with periods of comparative good health.

Stage 4:   Progression to AIDS, which may be diagnosed by a blood test to assess the condition of the immune system, or through a combination of major and minor signs of AIDS. The stage finishes with death, not from HIV infection itself, but from any or several of the opportunistic infections and cancers.

The time taken to move from Stage 1 to Stage 4 depends on factors specific to the individual, and the context in which he or she lives. People who are overworked, poorly nourished, and in poor health already have weakened immune systems, and so they progress more quickly than those who are well fed and in good health. Progression through the stages is also quicker in an environment where opportunistic diseases are common, and treatments for them are poor or entirely absent. As a result, the average time between HIV infection and the onset of AIDS is short in developing countries: some four to eight years. In richer nations the period is closer to eleven years and is now lengthening substantially, due to the widespread use of antiretroviral therapies. These drugs do not destroy HIV or cure AIDS, but they do delay or reverse the onset of AIDS, thereby improving quality of life and extending life expectancy.

Patterns of HIV infection

HIV/AIDS is unevenly spread not only in terms of geography but also in terms of other factors, which include age, sex, ethnicity, wealth, and occupation. In terms of age, HIV infection is generally concentrated among the most sexually active age groups, which also tend to be those age groups with the highest rates of injecting drug use. A universal pattern is that children and young people between the ages of 5 and 14 have low levels of infection. This is because most babies who are infected via their mothers are born in developing nations, and die before reaching the age of 5. Furthermore, infection through sexual activity or injecting drug use does not generally occur before the teenage years.

Sex is another factor: differing ratios between infected men and women result from the different patterns by which HIV is being transmitted. In sub-Saharan Africa and the Caribbean, where sexual activity between men and women is thought to be the main mode of transmission, the number of women who are infected equals or exceeds the number of infected men. In all other parts of the world, where injecting drug use and sex between men are the main modes of transmission, HIV-positive men outnumber HIV-positive women.

Some patterns of prevalence are related to ethnicity. For example, in the United States of America, the HIV epidemic is growing most rapidly among minority ethnic groups; African Americans form 12 per cent of the population, but about half of new HIV infections (UNAIDS 2003:28).

Finally, there is the factor of wealth and opportunity. Generally, while richer and more educated people are more likely to be infected in the early stages of a local epidemic, over time HIV tends to become concentrated among poorer people. HIV rates tend to be higher among women and men working in certain occupations which make them more susceptible to HIV infection. These include commercial sex work and jobs involving working away from home for long periods, such as mining, lorry driving, and service in the armed forces.

Of course, these factors do not exist in isolation. For example, in sub-Saharan Africa, analysis by sex and age reveals much higher rates of HIV infection among young women than among their male peers. Furthermore, the average age of death among HIV-positive women is around 25 years, whereas for men the average is 35 years.

Appendix 2 | AIDS work and development work: complementary strategies

Figure A.1 shows the positive relationships between development work with AIDS mainstreamed in it, HIV-prevention projects, and AIDS care and treatment.

It has long been known that efforts to prevent infection and to care for HIV-positive people reinforce each other. For example, education about HIV helps to reduce the numbers of people who need AIDS care and support, and also helps to challenge prejudice against HIV-positive people, including the belief that they do not deserve, or cannot benefit from, treatment. For its part, care and support for people with HIV/AIDS helps to prevent HIV infection by encouraging people who know that they are HIV-positive to practise safer sex, and by making the existence of AIDS more visible. The existence of treatment, and particularly of antiretroviral therapies, may also encourage more people to take an HIV test in the first place, again supporting prevention efforts by reducing denial and promoting positive living. (There are, however, some concerns that where effective antiretroviral treatment is widely available, it may actually undermine prevention efforts, because people assume that AIDS is curable.)

However, Figure A.1 also shows how both forms of AIDS work (HIV prevention and AIDS care) and development and humanitarian work reinforce each other. Successful AIDS-prevention programmes reduce the numbers of people who are HIV-infected, and so reduce the impacts of AIDS on development. Care, treatment, and support for people with AIDS can help to reduce the impacts of AIDS on individuals and their families, through extending lives, reducing wasteful expenditure on 'cures', improving productivity, and helping people to plan for their dependants' futures. In this way AIDS care and support can also help to reduce the numbers of households that slide into permanent destitution as a result of AIDS.

Equally, development and humanitarian work supports both kinds of AIDS work. Where development and humanitarian work leads to less poverty,

Figure A1 The positive interaction between AIDS work and development work

HIV Prevention

- Education about: modes of HIV transmission; means of preventing, or reducing the likelihood of, HIV infection; how HIV differs from AIDS
- Condom promotion and distribution
- STI treatment

Reduces susceptibility to infection, and increases effectiveness of prevention work:

- Better nutrition and health status ➡ lower biological susceptibility
- Less poverty and livelihoods insecurity ➡ less need to sell sex for survival
- Better health services ➡ greater access to STI treatment and condoms and less iatrogenic infection
- Greater gender equality ➡ women and men more able to act on prevention messages

Reduces numbers of people infected, therefore reduces all impacts of AIDS on development

Delayed sexual initiation and use of condoms also affect non-AIDS problems, such as unwanted pregnancies and associated school drop-outs, and STIs

Reduces numbers of people infected with HIV, and therefore numbers needing care

Education counteracts stigma by challenging misinformation about how HIV is transmitted

Promotes counselling, HIV testing, positive living, and seeking treatment. Involvement of HIV+ people may provide role models for this

Care and support to HIV+ people makes AIDS more visible, which counters denial in the general population

Voluntary counselling and testing enables people to discover their HIV status and encourages safer sex practices

Care and support helps HIV+ people to accept their condition and to live positively, including practising safer sex

Development

- Poverty alleviation
- Food and livelihoods security
- Health, water, and sanitation
- Education
- Humanitarian work following environmental crisis and conflict

AIDS Care

- Voluntary counselling and HIV testing
- Support for positive living, including material and spiritual support
- Treatment of opportunistic infections
- Anti-retroviral treatments
- Care when AIDS develops, at home or in a medical setting

Better health services ➡ strengthened systems for provision of counselling, testing, treatment, and care for people with AIDS

Less poverty and improved nutrition, water supply, and sanitation promote health of HIV+ people

Care and support reduce the impact of illness and death:

- Treatments enable HIV+ people to live and work longer
- Positive living reduces unproductive spending on 'cures', and encourages planning for death, e.g. making a will and arrangements for dependants

better standards of health, and greater gender equality, it reduces susceptibility to HIV infection, and so increases the effectiveness of prevention work. And where development work leads to better health services in general, it improves the delivery of HIV testing, AIDS care, and treatment. Furthermore, if development agencies raise standards of living in general (for example, through improved water and sanitation), then this benefits HIV+ people, helping (together with treatment and care) to extend their lives.

References

Barnett, T. and A. Whiteside (2002) *AIDS in the 21st Century: Disease and Globalization*, Basingstoke, UK: Palgrave Macmillan

Collins, J. and B. Rau (2000) 'AIDS in the Context of Development', UNRISD Programme on Social Policy and Development Paper number 4, Geneva: UNRISD and UNAIDS, www.unrisd.org

Donahue, J. (1998) 'Community-Based Economic Support for Households Affected by HIV/AIDS', Health Technical Services Project Report for TvT Associates, The Pragma Corporation, USAID HIV/AIDS Division, www.synergyaids.com

Donahue, J. (2002) 'Children, HIV/AIDS and Poverty in Southern Africa', unpublished paper presented to the Southern Africa Regional Poverty Network, 9–10 April 2002

FAO (2001) 'The Impact of HIV/AIDS on Food Security', meeting of Committee on World Food Security, Rome: FAO, www.fao.org

Ghana Ministry of Education (2002) 'Work Place Manual', HIV/AIDS Secretariat, Ministry of Education, Accra

Harvey, P. (2004) 'Appendix 9: The Issue of HIV/AIDS in the 2002/3 Relief Response in Southern Africa: a Background Discussion Paper for the DEC Evaluation', pp. 172–82 in Valid International (2004) 'A Stitch in Time?: Independent Evaluation of the Disasters Emergency Committee's Southern Africa Crisis Appeal July 2002 to June 2003', www.dec.org.uk

Holden, S. (2003) *AIDS on the Agenda: Adapting Development and Humanitarian Programmes to Meet the Challenge of HIV/AIDS*, Oxford: Oxfam GB

Loewenson, R. and A. Whiteside (2001) 'HIV/AIDS Implications for Poverty Reduction', New York: UNDP, www.undp.org

Piot, P. (2001) 'Facing the Challenge of AIDS', address by UNAIDS Executive Director to a UN Symposium on Nutrition and HIV/AIDS, Nairobi, 2 April 2001, www.unaids.org

Sphere Project (2000) *Humanitarian Charter and Minimum Standards in Disaster Response*, Oxford: Oxfam GB, www.sphereproject.org

Topouzis, D. (2001) 'Addressing the Impact of HIV/AIDS on Ministries of Agriculture: Focus on Eastern and Southern Africa', *Best Practice Digest*, Geneva: FAO and UNAIDS, www.unaids.org

Topouzis, D. and J. du Guerny (1999) 'Sustainable Agricultural/Rural Development and Vulnerability to the AIDS Epidemic', Geneva: FAO and UNAIDS, www.unaids.org

UNAIDS (2002) 'Report on the Global HIV/AIDS Epidemic', XIV International Conference on AIDS, Barcelona, 7–12 July 2002, Geneva: UNAIDS, www.unaids.org

UNAIDS (2003) 'AIDS Epidemic Update, December 2003', Geneva: UNAIDS/WHO, www.unaids.org

UNDP (2000) 'Botswana Human Development Report 2000', Gabarone: UNDP, www.undp.org

Index

direct
bio-medicine through health
services 47
dominant response 43
worthwhile but inadequate 116, 117
not suited to all development
organisations 36–7, 44
options for 56
problems faced by development
agencies 41–2
similarity to integrated AIDS work 16
antiretroviral therapies 10, 122Ap

behavioural factors 47
influencing HIV infection 44, *45*, *46*
bio-medical factors 47
influencing HIV infection 44, *45*, *46*
Botswana 32–3
boys 11, 12

capacity building
and participation 30
and training 76–7, 94–5, *100*, 110–-1
capacity maintenance 30
child mortality (under-five), affected by
AIDS 32
communities, AIDS-affected, focus of
development work 83
strengthening household safety nets 84
community research, external
mainstreaming 77–81, 91
community safety-nets 83
complementary partnerships 16, 19, 21,
22, 23, 56
in agricultural extension, CBO and
NGO 18
by micro-finance services NGO with
AIDS Support Organisation 20
crises, can lead to increased susceptibility
to HIV infection 8

development, seen as part of response to
HIV/AIDS 13
development agencies, problems faced
with AIDS work 41–2
development gains, reduced by AIDS 10

development and humanitarian agencies
47–9
external mainstreaming, ideal steps 110
implications for response to HIV and
AIDS summarised 49, 50
known negative effects of decision-
making 93
mainstreaming HIV/AIDS
beginning the process 53–5
key questions 52–3, *53*
options 55, *56*
may not achieve results proposed by
mainstreaming 38
should follow proposed measures
115–16
strategy and guiding principles 52–9
development and humanitarian work
and AIDS work, reinforcing each other
122Ap, *123Ap*, 124
attention to HIV/AIDS should be built
in 13–14
main differences in mainstreaming
HIV/AIDS 92–3
may exclude households affected by
AIDS 28–30
may increase susceptibility to HIV
infection 26–7, 104–5
may increase vulnerability to impacts
of AIDS 28
programmes relevant to acting against
AIDS before HIV-prevalence rises 105
well done, indirectly accts against HIV
and AIDS 104
see also development work;
humanitarian work
development organisations
advantages for those that mainstream
35–6
and AIDS impacts 34–5, 39
credibility and honesty of 37–8
not all equally suited for undertaking
AIDS work 36–7
workplace impacts of HIV/AIDS 33–4,
35
development problems, linked to
HIV/AIDS 2

strategy for 52–5, 56
supporting partners 101–2
where HIV-prevalence low 103–6
mainstreaming in humanitarian work
92–9, 100
adapting systems 99, 100
designing work which indirectly
addresses HIV and AIDS 97–9
'do no harm' approach 92–4, 100
emergency preparedness 95–6
summarised 99, 100
training and capacity building
94–5, 100
modifying ways in which
organisations function in context of
64–73
changing policy and practice 70–3
finance 72
learning about current impact of
AIDS 64–5
monitoring costs and trends 72–3
predicting impacts of AIDS,
analysing options for responding
66–9
terms, meanings and examples
summarised 23
and under-development 5–14
action on all influences needed
47–9
causes and consequences 6, 7, 10
deepening gender inequality
10–12, 13
household strategies in response to
9, 9
a medical and behavioural issue 5
a problem with no obvious solution 13
unevenly spread 121Ap
household coping strategies 9, 82–3, 84
household food insecurity, links with
AIDS 31
household safety-nets 83, 103, 105
households
access to water and sanitation
facilities, safety-net for poorest 88
AIDS-affected
effects on children 21

issues raised may not emerge
during project appraisals 38–9
learning about impacts of AIDS
from 41
may be excluded from
development and humanitarian
work 28–30
and micro-finance 20
under-represented in community
forums and in consultations 30
women and girls less likely to use
development opportunities 29
coping with shocks, implications for
development work 82–4
exclusion by judgemental staff 29
more vulnerable to AIDS though
development work 28
new and vulnerable forms may be
excluded by development agencies 29
poor 10, 105, 106
human-resources departments 71
*Humanitarian Charter and Minimum
Standards in Disaster Response*, Sphere
Project 96
humanitarian work
codes of conduct for workers 99
community research and consultation 96
designed to address HIV and AIDS
indirectly 97–9
decentralisation of tap stands,
latrines and washing facilities 97
distribution systems for food,
shelter materials and basic items
97–8
monitoring of work in camps 98
type and layout of accommodation
in camps 97
'do no harm' approach 92–4, 96, 97
external mainstreaming summarised
99, 100
inclusive 96
main differences from development
work 92–3
mainstreaming HIV/AIDS in, ideas
for 92–9, 100

infrastructure projects, unplanned effects
27
institutional audits 66
integrated AIDS work 15, 19, 20–1, 21, 23
internal mainstreaming 22, 23, 55, 56,
60–73, 74–5, 114, 115
AIDS impacts on the organisation
current, learning about 64–5, 74
predicted 66–9, 74
of AIDS-related issues in low-
prevalence settings 103–4
assessment of, confidentiality must be
maintained 112
by CBO, future effects of AIDS
considered 18
by development and humanitarian
agencies 47
by health promotion agency,
addressing an unsafe sex problem 19
by micro-financing services NGO 20
by a Ministry of Education 21
case for 33–6
devising/revising a workplace policy
62–4, 75
essential for all organisations 48
includes AIDS work with staff 16
modifying how organisations function
in context of AIDS 64–73, 75
raises issue of unsafe sex and sexual
bargaining 24
summary of key steps 74–5

labour loss due to AIDS 31
life expectancy 10, 32
livelihood security
becoming more fragile 31
improved by savings and credit
schemes 116
support from poverty-focused efforts
105–6

macro-environment 47
influencing HIV infection 45, 45, 46
mainstreaming 14, 24
arguments against 36–41
challenges to 106–13

challenges within 110–13
Collins and Rau quoted 117
examples 17–22
agricultural extension 18
education 20–1
health promotion 19
microfinance services NGO 19–20
water and sanitation services 21–2
importance where AIDS impact more
obvious 117
lack of clarity over meaning 107
lacks advocates 108
meaning of 15–17
more attractive proposition than
engaging in AIDS work 118
organisations lack resources to
undertake 108–9
short-term survival vs. long-term
strategy 109
something better than nothing 114
see also external mainstreaming;
internal mainstreaming
mainstreaming HIV/AIDS
the case for 3
externally and internally 15
guiding principles 57–9
ideas for 4
not an easy option 38
strategies for 52–5, 56
where AIDS-prevalence rates are low
103–6
see also external mainstreaming;
internal mainstreaming
Malawi 43–4
medical procedures, unsafe 11
medical treatment, for HIV infection 13
micro-enterprises, group-based 86–7
micro-environment 47
influencing HIV infection 44–5, 45, 46
micro-finance groups, AIDS-affected
members may be excluded 29
micro-finance projects/schemes 85–7, 116
micro-finance services NGO 19–20
migration, may increase susceptibility to
HIV infection 7, 27

shared learning, limited means of 112–13
social stigma, challenged 57
Southern Africa 5, 31
staff
awareness raising and basic training 55
clear terms and conditions of
employment 89
consultation with during
devising/revising workplace policy 63
facing up to AIDS as a personal issue,
helpful ideas 62
as focal points 54
and internal mainstreaming 38, 112
involved as active participants in
mainstreaming 57
motivated to look after own health 103–4
roles and responsibilities 89
support to reduce susceptibility to HIV,
and cope better with AIDS 60–4
susceptibility to HIV infection 70–1
STIs
rise in rates of 27
treatment in refugee camps 40
subsistence farming, suffers from cash
diversion to AIDS sufferers 31
susceptibility 34–5
may unintentionally be increased by
development work 25–6
to HIV infection
causes of 6B
increased through development
and humanitarian work 26–7

Thailand 31
training and capacity building
external mainstreaming 76–7
in humanitarian work 94–5
travel, regular, and casual sexual relations
70
twins, male and female, differing
consequences of AIDS 11–12

Uganda 31
UK, Department for International
Development, promoting
mainstreaming 118

UN General Assembly Special Session,
Declaration of Commitment 115
under-development 5–6, 37
unsafe sex 27
and development workers 26
girls pressured by male teachers 88
a problem for staff members 19
and sexual bargaining, between staff
and community members 24

violence, sexual and gender-based 12, 105
vulnerability 34–5
of agencies to AIDS impacts 47
may unintentionally be increased by
development work 25–6
to HIV infection 6B, 9–10
to impacts of AIDS, may be increased
by development and humanitarian
work 28

water and sanitation services
AIDS-affected households, prevented
from using 88
main project risk is potential for sexual
bargaining over access 87
NGO provision in a refugee camp 21–2
wealth, opportunity and HIV infection 121Ap
women and girls 105
in AIDS-affected households 29
may be subjected to demands for
sexual favours 79
in refugee camps, exposed to violence
98
rights to water and sanitation services
without sexual bargaining 87–8
suffer disproportionately in crises 8
trading sex for favours 117
workplace policy, creation of 62–4
appropriate level of benefits 62
changing policy and practice as result
of research 70–3
devising/revising a policy 63–4
all staff and managers to be aware
of final policy 63
cost-cutting possible in high HIV-
prevalence areas 63